T0301916

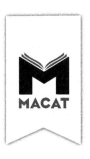

An Analysis of

Michel Foucault's

The History of Sexuality Vol. 1

The Will to Knowledge

Rachele Dini
and
Chiara Briganti

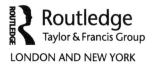

Routledge
Taylor & Francis Group

LONDON AND NEW YORK

Published by Macat International Ltd
24:13 Coda Centre, 189 Munster Road, London SW6 6AW.

Distributed exclusively by Routledge
2 Park Square, Milton Park, Abingdon, Oxon OX14 4RN
605 Third Avenue, New York, NY 10017

Routledge is an imprint of the Taylor & Francis Group, an informa business

Copyright © 2017 by Macat International Ltd
Macat International has asserted its right under the Copyright, Designs and Patents Act
1988 to be identified as the copyright holder of this work.

The print publication is protected by copyright. Prior to any prohibited reproduction, storage in
a retrieval system, distribution or transmission in any form or by any means, electronic, mechanical, recording or otherwise, permission should be obtained from the publisher or where
applicable a license permitting restricted copying in the United Kingdom should be obtained
from the Copyright Licensing Agency Ltd, Barnard's Inn, 86 Fetter Lane, London EC4A 1EN, UK.

The ePublication is protected by copyright and must not be copied, reproduced, transferred,
distributed, leased, licensed or publicly performed or used in any way except as specifically
permitted in writing by the publishers, as allowed under the terms and conditions under which
it was purchased, or as strictly permitted by applicable copyright law. Any unauthorised distribution or use of this text may be a direct infringement of the authors and the publishers' rights
and those responsible may be liable in law accordingly.

www.macat.com
info@macat.com

Cataloguing in Publication Data
A catalogue record for this book is available from the British Library.
Library of Congress Cataloguing-in-Publication Data is available upon request.
Cover illustration: Etienne Gilfillan

ISBN 978-1-912303-76-2 (hardback)
ISBN 978-1-912127-02-3 (paperback)
ISBN 978-1-912282-64-7 (e-book)

Notice
The information in this book is designed to orientate readers of the work under analysis,
to elucidate and contextualise its key ideas and themes, and to aid in the development
of critical thinking skills. It is not meant to be used, nor should it be used, as a
substitute for original thinking or in place of original writing or research. References and
notes are provided for informational purposes and their presence does not constitute
endorsement of the information or opinions therein. This book is presented solely for
educational purposes. It is sold on the understanding that the publisher is not engaged
to provide any scholarly advice. The publisher has made every effort to ensure that
this book is accurate and up-to-date, but makes no warranties or representations with
regard to the completeness or reliability of the information it contains. The information
and the opinions provided herein are not guaranteed or warranted to produce particular
results and may not be suitable for students of every ability. The publisher shall not be
liable for any loss, damage or disruption arising from any errors or omissions, or from
the use of this book, including, but not limited to, special, incidental, consequential or
other damages caused, or alleged to have been caused, directly or indirectly, by the
information contained within.

CONTENTS

THE MACAT LIBRARY

The Macat Library is a series of unique academic explorations of seminal works in the humanities and social sciences – books and papers that have had a significant and widely recognised impact on their disciplines. It has been created to serve as much more than just a summary of what lies between the covers of a great book. It illuminates and explores the influences on, ideas of, and impact of that book. Our goal is to offer a learning resource that encourages critical thinking and fosters a better, deeper understanding of important ideas.

Each publication is divided into three Sections: Influences, Ideas, and Impact. Each Section has four Modules. These explore every important facet of the work, and the responses to it.

This Section-Module structure makes a Macat Library book easy to use, but it has another important feature. Because each Macat book is written to the same format, it is possible (and encouraged!) to cross-reference multiple Macat books along the same lines of inquiry or research. This allows the reader to open up interesting interdisciplinary pathways.

To further aid your reading, lists of glossary terms and people mentioned are included at the end of this book (these are indicated by an asterisk [*] throughout) – as well as a list of works cited.

Macat has worked with the University of Cambridge to identify the elements of critical thinking and understand the ways in which six different skills combine to enable effective thinking.
Three allow us to fully understand a problem; three more give us the tools to solve it. Together, these six skills make up the **PACIER** model of critical thinking. They are:

ANALYSIS – understanding how an argument is built
EVALUATION – exploring the strengths and weaknesses of an argument
INTERPRETATION – understanding issues of meaning

CREATIVE THINKING – coming up with new ideas and fresh connections
PROBLEM-SOLVING – producing strong solutions
REASONING – creating strong arguments

To find out more, visit **WWW.MACAT.COM.**

CRITICAL THINKING AND *THE HISTORY OF SEXUALITY*

Primary critical thinking skill: CREATIVE THINKING
Secondary critical thinking skill: INTERPRETATION

Michel Foucault is famous as one of the 20th-century's most innovative and wide-ranging thinkers. The qualities that made him one of the most-read and influential theorists of the modern age find full expression in *The History of Sexuality*, the last project Foucault was able to complete before his death in 1984.

Central to Foucault's appeal is the creativity of his thought. Creative thinking takes many forms – from redefining an issue in a novel way to making unexpected and illuminating connections. Foucault's particular talent could perhaps best be described as turning questions inside out. In the case of sexuality, for instance, his interpretation of the historical evidence led him to argue that the sexual categories that we are used to (homosexual, lesbian, straight, and so on) are not "natural," but constructs that are products of the ways in which power and knowledge interact in society.

Such categories, Foucault continues, actually serve to produce the desires they seek to name. And their creation, in turn, is closely linked to the power that society exerts on those who belong to different sexual groups.

Foucault's ideas – familiar now – were so novel in their time that they proved highly challenging. But to see the world through Foucault's thought is to see it in a profoundly different and illuminating way – an example of creative thinking at its best.

ABOUT THE AUTHOR OF THE ORIGINAL WORK

Michel Foucault was born in 1926 into a wealthy and conservative French family. He studied philosophy, but being gay in a homophobic society took its toll, and after a suicide attempt in his early 20s, he was treated in a psychiatric hospital. Foucault is considered one of the most important modern thinkers. His analyses of the interplay of power, knowledge, and the makeup of the individual are considered key contributions to a wide range of academic fields, including sociology, history, and philosophy. Foucault died in 1984 at the age of 57.

ABOUT THE AUTHORS OF THE ANALYSIS

Dr Rachele Dini studied at Cambridge, King's College London and University College London. Much of her current work focuses on the representation of production and consumption in modern and contemporary Anglo-American fiction. She has taught at Cambridge and for the Foundation for International Education, and is now Ledturer in English at the University of Roehampton. Her first monograph, *Consumerism, Waste and Re-use in Twentieth-century Fiction: Legacies of the Avant-Garde*, was published by Palgrave Macmillan in 2016.

Dr Chiara Briganti was a professor of English Literature and Gender Studies at Carleton College, for many years, and is now a visiting research fellow at King's College London. Dr Briganti is co-author, of *Domestic Modernism, the Interwar Novel*, and *E.H.Young* and *The Domestic Space Reader* (University of Toronto Press, 2013).

ABOUT MACAT

GREAT WORKS FOR CRITICAL THINKING

Macat is focused on making the ideas of the world's great thinkers accessible and comprehensible to everybody, everywhere, in ways that promote the development of enhanced critical thinking skills.

It works with leading academics from the world's top universities to produce new analyses that focus on the ideas and the impact of the most influential works ever written across a wide variety of academic disciplines. Each of the works that sit at the heart of its growing library is an enduring example of great thinking. But by setting them in context – and looking at the influences that shaped their authors, as well as the responses they provoked – Macat encourages readers to look at these classics and game-changers with fresh eyes. Readers learn to think, engage and challenge their ideas, rather than simply accepting them.

'Macat offers an amazing first-of-its-kind tool for interdisciplinary learning and research. Its focus on works that transformed their disciplines and its rigorous approach, drawing on the world's leading experts and educational institutions, opens up a world-class education to anyone.'

Andreas Schleicher
Director for Education and Skills, Organisation for Economic Co-operation and Development

'Macat is taking on some of the major challenges in university education ... They have drawn together a strong team of active academics who are producing teaching materials that are novel in the breadth of their approach.'

Prof Lord Broers,
former Vice-Chancellor of the University of Cambridge

'The Macat vision is exceptionally exciting. It focuses upon new modes of learning which analyse and explain seminal texts which have profoundly influenced world thinking and so social and economic development. It promotes the kind of critical thinking which is essential for any society and economy.
This is the learning of the future.'

Rt Hon Charles Clarke, former UK Secretary of State for Education

'The Macat analyses provide immediate access to the critical conversation surrounding the books that have shaped their respective discipline, which will make them an invaluable resource to all of those, students and teachers, working in the field.'

Professor William Tronzo, University of California at San Diego

WAYS IN TO THE TEXT

KEY POINTS

- Michel Foucault is among the twentieth century's most influential social scientists; he wrote widely on the relationship between knowledge and power.

- Foucault's *The History of Sexuality Vol. 1* (1976) challenged then-widespread views about sexuality and sexual repression, and offered a new approach to understanding the relationship between sexuality, knowledge, and power.

- *The History of Sexuality* changed the way scholars talked about sex and sexuality, and paved the way for a host of new academic disciplines, including gender studies* (inquiry into the ways that gender—the sum of attributes considered to represent identities such as "male" or "female"—are constituted by society) and queer theory* (an approach to cultural analysis that begins by acknowledging the instability and uncertainty of sexual identity and knowledge itself).

Who Is Michel Foucault?

Michel Foucault (1926–84), the author of *The History of Sexuality Vol. 1: The Will to Knowledge*, was a French philosopher, historian, and writer. He is best known as the author of *The Birth of the Clinic* (1963) (a study of the history of medicine), of *Madness and Civilization* (1964), and of a study of the modern prison, *Discipline and Punish* (1975). His

History of Sexuality was originally intended as the first of a six-volume examination of how sex has been understood throughout history.

Foucault was interested in how different systems of knowledge originate, and how knowledge is used to control, regulate, and even shape people's identities. His work explores the nature of the power associated with knowledge, and how knowledge systems evolve over time.

In 1976, when he published *Sexuality Vol. 1*, Foucault was already a respected intellectual with a global reputation. In 1969 he was appointed professor at the *Collège de France*, a prestigious higher education institution in Paris (professorships there are reserved for highly established academics). He chose for himself the title Historian of Systems of Thought. As a professor, Foucault was responsible for giving an annual series of lectures on the theme of his choice. One of them was the subject that became the first volume of his *History of Sexuality*. Foucault died of an AIDS*-related illness in 1984, shortly after the publication of *Vol. 2** and *Vol. 3*.*

What Does *The History of Sexuality* Say?

Foucault looks at the ways in which sex has been talked about in the modern Western world. Since the Middle Ages* (approximately the sixth to the fourteenth centuries), he claims that Western societies have increasingly turned to the practice of Roman Catholic* confession* as a means of putting sexual practices and desires into words (in confession, Roman Catholic Christians confess their sins to a priest in exchange for forgiveness). This argument went against a commonly held view among scholars of his time that sex—particularly in the nineteenth century—was not talked about, and that the Church and the state tried to prevent all mention of it.

Foucault also believes that calls for sexual liberation are related to the fact that sex has been talked about a great deal in modern times. He makes his argument in contrast to what he calls the "repressive hypothesis."* According to this theory, which was often behind the loud calls for sexual liberation in the 1960s and 1970s, natural expressions of sexuality have been repressed and silenced by the bourgeoisie* (the rich and powerful class of business owners). Foucault says this idea developed from Victorian* attitudes to sex (the straightlaced approach that characterized the reign of Britain's Queen Victoria from 1837 to 1901), which were commonly seen as having been restricted and repressed.

Foucault contrasts the open attitudes toward sex of the seventeenth century with those of the Victorian period, but he maintains that, contrary to what people believed, the Victorians did not hide sex behind closed doors. Although they did try to stop talk about sex, in practice they were not very successful. This is a valuable part of Foucault's analysis. He maintains that during the eighteenth and nineteenth centuries sex was talked about a lot, and was even turned into an object of scientific study. A complex scientific conversation arose around sexuality that led to the identification of certain pathologies* (or types of disorders), such as the homosexual,* the hysterical* woman, or the masturbating child. This information was then used to establish definitions and theories about normal and abnormal behavior and, in turn, to create laws to regulate sexuality.

However, according to Foucault, this discourse (that is, discussion) around sex accepted various sexualities and treated them as legitimate. Moreover, this attitude was not directly imposed on the lower classes (the wage earners and small farmers) by the dominant class (the bourgeoisie or business owners). Instead, it was first developed to reassure the dominant class of its superiority before spreading to the lower classes.

By investigating sexual history and theory, Foucault concludes that power in modern societies is not enforced so much by suppression or direct domination (the use of force and violence). Instead, power over the population is exercised through complex and scattered techniques and mechanisms, mainly involving the production of knowledge, scientific or otherwise.

Why Does *The History of Sexuality* Matter?

Sexuality Vol. 1 changed the way scholars thought about sex and sexuality, power, and knowledge. It suggested a whole new approach to the study of sexuality that favored historical analysis rather than psychoanalysis,* (a therapeutic and theoretical approach to the unconscious mind developed by the Austrian thinker Sigmund Freud* in the late nineteenth century). It also introduced a new way of thinking about sex and power that complicated the simplistic explanations that were popular at the time.

The 1960s saw a profound change in attitudes toward sex. Those who supported sexual liberation, along with social science* and humanities* scholars, tended to see a conflict between an individual's instinctive desires and the various authorities that tried to limit it ("humanities" here refers to academic disciplines relating to the study of human culture, such as history and literature). Such authorities could be the government, the Church, or even a repressive parent or spouse. Those who shared this view thought that sexual liberation would only come about by allowing people to follow their sexual desires without being prevented by laws or social customs.

Foucault challenged this view, maintaining that both sexuality and power are far more complex than a strict division between instinct and authority would suggest. In making this claim, he opened up a new way of thinking about sex and sexuality, and paved the way for new disciplines such as gender and sexuality studies,* and new ideas such as queer theory, which helped broaden the debate around the social role of sex. The text continues to be an important work for anyone interested in gender and sexuality, and is significant for those seeking to understand Foucault's overall thinking.

SECTION 1
INFLUENCES

MODULE 1
THE AUTHOR AND THE
HISTORICAL CONTEXT

KEY POINTS

- *The History of Sexuality Vol. 1* was a groundbreaking work of philosophical and cultural criticism that changed the way scholars thought about sexuality and power.

- Foucault was shaped by his conservative upbringing and postwar France's repressive ideas about sexuality; in the 1960s and 1970s he was active in left-wing movements.

- While his own homosexuality* and liberal* views were at odds with the culture of his time, Foucault's ideas on sexuality were also at odds with those of the French left.

Why Read This Text?

Michel Foucault's *The History of Sexuality Vol. 1: The Will to Knowledge* is a study of the evolution of cultural ideas about sex. It examines how the idea of sexuality was used to regulate, control, and rule. Foucault argues that, since the end of the seventeenth century, the discussion of sex in Western culture grew across different branches of science, such as biology* (the study of living things), psychiatry* (the study and treatment of mental disorders), and pedagogy* (teaching). As an object of scientific knowledge, sexual preferences came to be seen as a problem of "truth" that could reveal something about a person's identity.

The core question Foucault sets out to answer is: "Why do we say, with so much passion and so much resentment against our most recent past, against our present, and against ourselves, that we are repressed?"[1] Throughout the book, and the following two volumes of the series,

❝ Since the end of the sixteenth century, the 'putting into discourse of sex,' far from undergoing a process of restriction, on the contrary has been subjected to a mechanism of increasing incitement … the will to knowledge has not come to a halt in the face of a taboo that must not be lifted, but has persisted in constituting—despite many mistakes, of course—a science of sexuality. ❞

Michel Foucault, *The History of Sexuality Vol. 1: The Will to Knowledge*

Foucault argues that a will to know and speak about sex affects the ways that our societies understand sexual desires and practices.

Sexuality Vol. 1 broke new ground. It changed the way scholars thought about sexuality and power. It also drew attention to the way that, over the centuries, rules about sex have been used to regulate citizens' behavior and uphold state power. Foucault came up with a new way of understanding the concept of power: it was, he said, "polymorphous"*—that is, something that takes many shapes, and invades all aspects of life, rather than something imposed by one ruler.

Author's Life

Michel Foucault was born in 1926 into an upper-middle class family in Poitiers, France. Resisting expectations to become a doctor like his father, he enrolled in the Lycée Henri-IV, a highly regarded secondary school in Paris, where he studied philosophy under the famous philosopher Jean Hyppolite.* [2] He then entered the *École Normale Supérieure d'Ulm* (ENS), the most prestigious French university for the humanities,* where he studied under the Marxist* philosopher Louis Althusser* (Marxism is a method of social and historical analysis founded on the thought of the nineteenth-century political philosopher Karl Marx).* He graduated with a degree in psychological sciences in 1948, and with a second degree in philosophy in 1951. While studying philosophy, he worked with the renowned phenomenologist* Maurice Merleau-Ponty.* (Phenomenology is the branch of philosophy that studies the structures that inform our experience and our consciousness of the world around us, and the role that perception plays in the way we relate to the world.)

Foucault openly stated that his books were not only influenced by the scholars he studied, but also by his personal experiences. Although his father came from a strict Roman Catholic* background (Roman Catholicism being the largest branch of the Christian faith), Foucault was not religious, and he was suspicious of beliefs that attempted to interpret the world in its entirety. This can, in part, explain his lasting concern with knowledge and power. Perhaps more importantly, as a gay man living in conservative postwar France, Foucault experienced firsthand an oppressive heteronormative* culture (a culture that accepts only heterosexuality* as the norm, and condemns homosexuality). Foucault attempted suicide in 1948 and was hospitalized in a psychiatric institution in Paris. His doctors diagnosed his later attempts to kill himself as reactions to the social stigma and shame attached to being openly gay.

At the time Foucault was writing *Sexuality Vol. 1*, he had already been appointed as a professor at the highly respected *Collège de France*, holding one of the highest academic positions in the country. The year following publication, he was invited to consult with the French government on changes to the laws dealing with rape.[3] Foucault was also politically active in left-wing movements throughout the 1970s. Most notably, he was a member of *Groupe d'Information sur les Prisons* (*Prison Information Group**), a group that fought for inmates' rights and distributed information about prisons. Foucault died in 1984 in Paris from an HIV*-related disease.

Author's Background

Foucault's concerns in *Sexuality Vol. 1,* as well as in his other works, were very much of their time. Although France in the 1970s was relatively stable, the previous decade had seen intense social upheaval. The country had endured several bitter conflicts, including opposition to its bloody but ultimately unsuccessful wars to keep its colonies (Vietnam won independence in 1954 but French activists laid the blame for the subsequent Vietnam War* on France's legacy in the area; Algeria won its independence in 1962), and what students saw as the elitism of the education system. There was also widespread anticapitalist* sentiment that gave rise to strikes and occupations across the land (capitalism is the social and economic system dominant in the West and increasingly throughout the world, in which trade and industry are conducted for private profit). This unrest climaxed with the events of May 1968,* during which students occupied the Sorbonne university, a prestigious and notably old seat of learning in Paris, to oppose the capitalist system and traditional values.

The students' occupation inspired the largest workers' strike the country had ever seen, during which the French economy effectively ground to a halt. Both the student occupation and the strike were finally put down with police force, and the events did little to change France's political structure. However, those two weeks of unrest came to be seen as a watershed moment. The women's rights movement in France began immediately after the events of 1968, and French feminism* and interest in sexuality as a concept grew over the course of the 1970s (feminism denotes the intellectual and political currents associated with the struggle for equality between the sexes).

This background provides important insight into the origins of Foucault's work. In particular, although Foucault participated in many of the leftist* movements of the 1960s, *Sexuality Vol. 1* does not endorse the views of the left concerning sex and sexuality. His objective in the book was in fact to challenge the arguments for sexual

17

liberation common among leftist thinkers. The discussion of the period centered on the tension between people's instinctual sexual drives and the state powers or capitalist forces that sought to repress them. Foucault argued that this picture of oppressed and oppressors was overly simplistic, and he sought to complicate it.

NOTES

1   Michel Foucault, *The History of Sexuality Vol. 1: The Will to Knowledge*, trans. Robert Hurley (London: Penguin Books, 1998), 8–9.

2   Daniel Defert, "Chronology," in *A Companion to Foucault*, eds. Christopher Falzon et al. (Chichester: Wiley & Sons, 2013), 11.

3   See Monique Plaza, "Our Costs and Their Benefits," in *Sex in Question: French Materialist Feminism*, eds. Diana Leonard and Lisa Adkins (London: Taylor & Francis, 1996), 184.

MODULE 2
ACADEMIC CONTEXT

KEY POINTS

- Foucault challenged the popular use of psychoanalytic* ideas to explain sexuality, rejecting the idea that people are born with their sexuality, and proposing that it is a result of social conditions.

- Foucault was associated with the structuralist* and poststructuralist* schools of thought, though he never accepted being part of either movement. (Structuralism and poststructuralism are approaches to the analysis of culture that differ on matters such as the extent to which we can be certain of objective knowledge.)

- Foucault was greatly influenced by the nineteenth-century German philosopher Friedrich Nietzsche.*

The Work in its Context

After May 1968* Michel Foucault's *The History of Sexuality Vol. 1: The Will to Knowledge* entered into the debates taking place both in intellectual circles and in society in general (May 1968 was a time of radical social activism in Europe and the United States). In that era, the 1960s and 1970s, Western academic discussions of sex and sexuality were largely influenced by psychoanalytic thought.

Psychoanalysis began at the end of the nineteenth century. It was first developed by the Austrian neurologist* Sigmund Freud, who viewed a person's identity as formed by their unconscious desires and repressed childhood memories—memories people force themselves to forget since society considers them unacceptable (e.g., sexual love for a parent or the sight of one's own parents having sex). Freud argued that an individual's sexual identity was shaped by these experiences. In

❝ What is peculiar to modern societies, in fact, is not that they consigned sex to a shadow existence, but that they dedicated themselves to speaking of it *ad infinitum*, while exploiting it as *the* secret.❞

Michel Foucault, *The History of Sexuality Vol. 1: The Will to Knowledge*

the 1960s and 1970s, social scientists, such as the German American philosopher Herbert Marcuse* and the Austrian psychoanalyst Wilhelm Reich,* introduced psychoanalytic concepts into their work. Foucault challenged their positions by offering a new way of thinking of sexuality, seeing it as an effect of social conditioning and not as something you are simply born with.

Foucault challenged psychoanalytic thought by claiming that a person's sexual orientation or preference does not come so much from instinct and unconscious urges as from ideals learned in society. He writes that sexuality is organized around two ideas: "deviant" and "normal" sexual behaviors. For Foucault, this distinction helps separate sexual activities that a particular society considers acceptable (such as heterosexual,* reproductive sex within marriage) from those considered unacceptable (such as homosexual* activity and extramarital sex). Foucault argues that there is nothing natural or universal about these codes of behavior. Since society's view of what is deviant and what is considered normal changes over time, sexuality does as well. Put differently, sexuality is a product of changing sociohistorical circumstances and not unconscious drives, as claimed by psychoanalysis.

Moreover, Foucault argued that the psychoanalytic focus on talking about sexual repression was just another product of modern mechanisms of power. Psychoanalysis might claim that talking about sex openly could help unlock an individual's repressed experiences, but Foucault argued this view was itself a form of control, and not so different from the methods used by Victorian doctors to "cure" people of their sexual "perversions." The interest in talking about sex as a way to combat repression was common in France in the aftermath of May 1968. Foucault's resistance to such an approach was highly original.

Overview of the Field

As well as psychoanalysis, two other schools of thought—structuralism and poststructuralism—greatly influenced the course of twentieth-century thinking in the humanities* and social sciences,* and were also closely related to Foucault's work. In fact, his three-volume *History of Sexuality* (as well as his other writings) has been labeled structuralist and poststructuralist, even though Foucault himself resisted such labels.

Structuralism was developed after World War I* (1914–18) by scholars such as the Swiss linguist* Ferdinand de Saussure* and, later, the French anthropologist* Claude Lévi-Strauss* and the French philosopher Louis Althusser*—Foucault's teacher and a formative influence on his thinking. (Linguistics is the study of the nature and functioning of language, while anthropology is the study of human beings, especially our cultures, beliefs, and societies.) These thinkers believed that all culture is constructed—that is, the product of laws and unwritten rules that govern how people behave and what they believe. To understand any single element of culture, it was assumed, one must examine the institutions or whole social system of which it is a part.

Foucault's central point in *The History of Sexuality*—that sexuality is constructed by each society—can be understood as a structuralist approach. According to this view, all elements of culture exist—and are shaped by—their relation to larger ideas, institutions, and systems of their society.[1] In the same way, structuralism sees sexuality as something that is not the same for all societies, but rather depends on historical and cultural circumstances.

Poststructuralism was a movement that developed out of structuralism in the 1960s and 1970s, derived from the work of mostly

French theorists and philosophers, such as Jacques Derrida.* These scholars regarded our understanding of social structures and categories as naturally unstable—that is, subject to change, and not very valid. They claimed that because all individuals are a product of their historical context, and are participants in their culture, no one could really examine *anything* "objectively," and without bias. Any scholar who examines a cultural artifact (anything made by people—and reflecting their culture) must, therefore, recognize that their own situation and background will to some extent influence their analysis. In this way, *The History of Sexuality* can also be read as a poststructuralist work in that its central aim is to disturb given categories and disprove stable definitions.[2]

While Foucault is often associated with poststructuralism, he was not a committed member of any particular school of thought. His historical approach and method is associated with the Annales School,* (an influential French school of historical inquiry that *focused on social rather than diplomatic or political issues in studying history),* but he never clearly stated that he was part of it.

Academic Influences

Foucault's work is highly indebted to the nineteenth-century German philosopher Friedrich Nietzsche. The approach that Foucault used in *Sexuality Vol. 1*, which he called "genealogical* critique," owes much to Nietzsche's *On the Genealogy of Morals** (1887).[3]

Genealogy, in philosophy, refers to the analysis of a historical period's different belief systems alongside each other, rather than individually. Rather than focusing on the origins of these systems, genealogy is interested in the conditions that allow them to exist (for example, the laws in place at the time). Foucault used this term to describe his own approach to historical analysis, which assumed all truths to be questionable and history itself to be a construct that can be endlessly revised as each generation offers a different viewpoint on the past that often contradicts the ideas of the generation before. *Sexuality Vol. 1*'s subtitle *The Will to Knowledge* refers to Nietzsche's "will to power,"* a term he used to describe what he believed was the motivating force in humans: ambition and the desire to achieve the highest possible position available to them. It also reflects Foucault's main aim: to analyze how the will to know and speak about sexuality forms itself and how it affects the ways our societies understand sexual practices.

Foucault admitted that Nietzsche was among his greatest influences, stating, "if I wanted to be pretentious, I would use 'the genealogy of morals' as the general title of what I am doing."[4] More generally, Foucault's interest in how scientists have examined sexuality as an object of knowledge reflects his lifelong aim to question modern structures and institutions.

NOTES

1 Hubert L. Dreyfus and Paul Rabinow, eds., *Michel Foucault: Beyond Structuralism and Hermeneutics* (Chicago: University of Chicago Press, 1983); David H. J. Larmour et al., "Situating the *History of Sexuality*," in *Rethinking Sexuality: Foucault and Classical Antiquity,* eds. David H. J. Larmour et al., (Princeton, New Jersey: Princeton University Press, 1998), 3–41.

2 See Nikki Sullivan, *A Critical Introduction to Queer Theory* (New York: NYU Press, 2003), 40.

3 See Friedrich Nietzsche, *On the Genealogy of Morals and Ecce Homo* (New York: Random House, 2010).

4 Alan D. Schrift, *Nietzsche's French Legacy: A Genealogy of Poststructuralism* (London: Routledge, 1995), 33.

MODULE 3
THE PROBLEM

KEY POINTS

- *Sexuality Vol. 1* challenged the way scholars thought about sex, sexuality, and power, and challenged common ideas about sexuality's role in nineteenth-century society.

- Foucault's text rejected the theoretical approach founded on the work of the nineteenth-century political philosopher Karl Marx* and the founder of psychoanalysis* Sigmund Freud* that dominated academic thought in his field in the 1960s and 1970s.

- *Sexuality Vol. 1* offered a new way of thinking about repression and power, arguing against the ideas of scholars such as the German American cultural critic Herbert Marcuse,* and claiming that power cannot be located in one single place or person.

Core Question

Michel Foucault's *The History of Sexuality Vol. 1: The Will to Knowledge* challenged the way sexuality was understood both within the intellectual circles of his time, and by the public at large. The book's core question is: "Why does a society like ours speak so openly about sexual repression?" The way Foucault approached it was highly original. He developed an entirely new way of thinking about sexuality and power that went against current scholarship.

Sexuality Vol. 1 sought to demonstrate that sexuality is not simply something that the dominant classes (that is, the rich and powerful) of a society look to repress in the lower classes—a view held by many humanities* and social science* scholars during the 1960s and 1970s. Foucault disputes what he calls this "repressive hypothesis."* The

❝ [Modernity* made] the flesh into the root of all evil, shifting the most important moment of transgression from the act itself to the stirrings—so difficult to perceive and formulate—of desire. For this was an evil that afflicted the whole man, and in the most secret of forms. **❞**

Michel Foucault, *The History of Sexuality Vol. 1: The Will to Knowledge*

repressive hypothesis assumes that power, whether in the form of law or of bourgeois* (middle-class) society, in general represses sexuality. For instance, it is considered improper to talk about sex openly, and it is assumed that only the lower classes satisfy their sexual appetites without restraint. In this sense, sexual liberation will come only if we radically break free from all these restrictions on sexuality. According to these views, power works solely in negative terms: it represses and prohibits instinctive sexual drives.

Foucault rejected this position. He argued instead that power is also positive and productive in the sense that it shapes the way we see the world, including our desires and preferences.

The text challenged the social movements of the 1960s and 1970s that, following the repressive hypothesis, claimed they were liberating the public from repressive attitudes left over from the nineteenth century. By maintaining that nineteenth-century views on sexuality were in fact more complex than scholars thought, Foucault suggested that the arguments of left-wing activists were overly simple and historically inaccurate.

The Participants

Foucault's text was partly a critique of Freudo-Marxism,* an approach to cultural analysis drawing on Sigmund Freud's psychoanalysis and Karl Marx's critique of the social and economic system of capitalism.*

25

Freudian psychoanalysis sees culture as a product of people's actions and of our unconscious desires and suppressed urges. Marxist criticism sees culture in terms of the conflicts between people of different socioeconomic classes.

Viewed through the lens of Freudo-Marxism, sexuality is, above all, a tool for oppression. The upper classes of society decide what is proper and then use these rules to dominate the lower classes, while individuals face the conflict between their inner desires and society's ideas of what is acceptable. This idea can be attributed to the German psychoanalyst Wilhelm Reich.* In his theory of "sexual repression" Reich suggests that repression is a necessary part of capitalist exploitation. He argues that "the compulsion to control one's sexuality … leads to the development of pathologic [diseased], emotionally tinged notions of honor and duty, bravery and self-control."[1] In Reich's view, repression could even make the masses ready to accept authoritarian forms of rule—systems in which personal liberty is sacrificed to governmental authority.

Foucault questioned Reich's views, but was especially interested in Reich's urge to speak about sexual repression. For Foucault, the efforts of psychiatrists and biologists to put sexuality into words showed their own biases. Toward the end of *Sexuality Vol. 1* he notes, "The fact that so many things were able to change in the sexual behavior of Western societies [the loosening of attitudes toward sex, aided by the widespread availability of the 'pill' and other birth-control methods, for example] without any of the promises or political conditions predicted by Reich being realized is sufficient proof that this whole sexual 'revolution,' this whole 'anti-repressive' struggle, represented nothing more, but nothing less—and its importance is undeniable—than a tactical shift and reversal in the great deployment of sexuality."[2]

By this, Foucault meant that although the sexual revolution was undeniably important, it was important for different reasons from those given to it by the political left. He saw it as a fascinating example of how different interest groups (scientific institutions, political parties, and so on) developed ideas about sex to further their own aims. Where "the great deployment of sexuality" in the Victorian era served to diagnose mental illnesses and restrict behavior, in the 1960s it became a means to take down these restrictions. For Foucault, the interesting thing is the consistency with which different institutions, with often opposing views, have used sexuality—that is, the discussion of sex—to advance their political agenda.

Foucault saw Reich as one of the strongest promoters of the repressive hypothesis and was very skeptical of the whole idea of sexual or other liberation. Foucault took a position against the Freudo-Marxist approaches that largely shaped the intellectual debates of his time and presented new ideas to replace those he was critiquing. His text set out to show how people in the nineteenth century *actually* thought about sex and sexuality, and, more broadly, to prove that power does not work the way many assume.

The Contemporary Debate

Sexuality Vol. 1 can also be seen to target the American-based German philosopher Herbert Marcuse. Although Marcuse's name is not directly mentioned anywhere in the text, Foucault often mentioned him in interviews in which he discussed his "repressive hypothesis." For example, in an interview he gave a year before *Sexuality Vol. 1* was published, Foucault distanced himself "from para-Marxists like Marcuse who give the notion of repression an exaggerated role."[3]

In the book itself, Foucault's rejection of Marcuse's ideas is clear when he talks about power. One of Marcuse's central and most influential ideas was the concept of the "great refusal."* He defined this as "the protest against unnecessary repression, the struggle for the ultimate form of freedom—'to live without anxiety'."[4] In other words, to live freely one must reject all forms of repression, and oppose the efforts of those in power to dictate how one should behave or what o   n   e

should believe.

In contrast to Marcuse, Foucault claims that power does not reside in a single person or place, whose influence one can resist. Instead, power is multidimensional, distributed across relations and networks. As he puts it in *Sexuality Vol. 1*, "there is no single locus of great Refusal, no soul of revolt, source of all rebellions, or pure law of the revolutionary."[5] This statement clearly suggests a critique of Marcuse's idea. Because power is spread out, rejecting power is much more complicated than Marcuse's theory suggests, for it involves countering more than the authority of a single person (a king, one's boss) or institution (the government, a company).

NOTES

1   Wilhelm Reich, (New York: Farrar, Straus & Giroux, 1970), 54.

2   Michel Foucault, *The History of Sexuality Vol. 1: The Will to Knowledge,* trans. Robert Hurley (London: Penguin Books, 1998), 131.

3   Michel Foucault, *Power/Knowledge: Selected Interviews and Other Writings, 1972–1977,* ed. Colin Gordon, trans. Colin Gordon et al. (New York: Random House, Inc., 1980), 59.

4   Herbert Marcuse, (Beacon Press, 1974 [1955]), 149–50.

5   Foucault, *Sexuality Vol. 1*, 95–6.

MODULE 4
THE AUTHOR'S CONTRIBUTION

KEY POINTS

- Foucault put forward an original theory of power as both dispersed and productive—having the capacity to *construct* desires, identities, and pleasures, rather than just repress them.

- He focused on the body, and not the individual, as the place where control over people is exercised.

- *Sexuality Vol. 1* was intended to be the first of six volumes that would analyze sexuality's role throughout the ages; *Vol. 1* looked at the nineteenth century, *Vol. 2** examined sexuality in ancient Greece, and *Vol. 3** considered ancient Rome.

Author's Aims

Michel Foucault's *The History of Sexuality Vol. 1: The Will to Knowledge* aimed to achieve three goals: to challenge the "repressive hypothesis,"* to show that sex from the late seventeenth century onwards was examined as an object of scientific analysis, and to advance a new theory about how power operates.

Foucault sought to show that experts such as psychologists,* biologists,* medical doctors, demographers* (those analyzing the ways in which a certain society is made up statistically) from the late seventeenth century onwards viewed sex as a problem of "truth"—a matter to be examined, written about, and understood. Related to this, he aimed to demonstrate that the modern view of eighteenth- and nineteenth-century bourgeois* society as repressive was part of the same dominant narrative that had sought to first repress sexuality. Put differently, he argued that this "knowledge" of a sexually repressive

29

> 66 Sexuality must not be thought of as a kind of natural given which power tries to hold in check, or as an obscure domain which knowledge tries gradually to uncover. It is the name that can be given to a historical construct. 99

Michel Foucault, *The History of Sexuality Vol. 1: The Will to Knowledge*

history was, itself, constructed: "Why do we say, with so much passion and so much resentment against our most recent past, against our present, and against ourselves, that we are repressed?"[1]

Foucault put forward an original theory of power as something dispersed, rather than located in any one person or place. By exploring how nineteenth-century thinkers studied sex, Foucault aimed to show that power is not only repressive, it is also productive, and has the capacity to *construct* desires, identities, and pleasures rather than just repress them. In short, Foucault set out to define "the regime of power-knowledge-pleasure that sustains the discourse on human sexuality in our part of the world."[2]

Approach

Foucault intended Sexuality Vol. 1 to be the first of a six-volume work that would examine how sexuality was represented, and the role it played, throughout history. In *Vol. 1*, Foucault examines, compares, and contrasts theological,* psychiatric,* and medical texts and practices from the Middle Ages* to the nineteenth century in order to understand how views on sexuality changed in the eighteenth and nineteenth centuries.

Foucault approaches his analysis of the theoretical and practical context of sexuality by focusing on the body as the location of control over individuals. This focus on the body, instead of on the individual, is significant. The individual is not a basic, stable entity that those in power can target. Foucault wants to avoid focusing on any particular party in power relations. He emphasizes that it is not just institutions that oppress people, but that the most commonplace relations also influence institutions. That is, there is no main agent—active force— exercising power. Power, Foucault says, works bottom up as much as top down.

Contribution in Context

Because Foucault died from an HIV*-related illness shortly after the publication of *Vols. 2* and *3*, it is difficult to say how close he came to achieving his original aims. It is similarly impossible to know how our opinion of his work, and our approach to his entire output, would be different had all six volumes of *The History of Sexuality* been completed. The delay in the publication of *Vols. 2* and *3* (they appeared eight years after the first volume) can be read as evidence that he lost interest in the project, or that he reached some sort of intellectual stalemate. However, Foucault's delay can also point to troubles he had with his publishers.[3] Although Foucault's initial aim for the project has only been partly realized, the volumes he managed to publish clearly changed the way scholars thought about sex. They also contributed to the discussion of power relations and knowledge initiated by his earlier works.

Although the books share some of the same concerns—notably the relationship between sexuality and power, the regulation of desire, and the socially constructed nature of the body—*Vol. 2* and *Vol. 3* of *The History of Sexuality* take a rather different approach to *Vol. 1*. In *Vol. 2,* Foucault considers the role of erotic pleasure across ancient Greek culture, focusing on its depiction in numerous ancient Greek texts. In *Vol. 3*, he examines sexuality's role in ancient Rome, focusing on the meditations on sex by philosophers such as Seneca,* Plutarch* and Epictetus* to understand how views of sex changed over the course of the Roman Empire. Both volumes seek to understand the reasons behind Western culture's tendency to judge sexuality in moral terms, and to regulate it far more than other physical appetites such as hunger, sleep, or aggression.

NOTES

1   Michel Foucault, *The History of Sexuality Vol. 1: The Will to Knowledge,* trans. Robert Hurley (London: Penguin Books, 1998), 8–9.

2   Foucault, *Sexuality Vol. 1,* 11.

3   See Daniel Defert, "Chronology," in *A Companion to Foucault*, eds. Christopher Falzon et al. (Chichester: Wiley & Sons, 2013), 60.

SECTION 2
IDEAS

MODULE 5
MAIN IDEAS

KEY POINTS

- *Sexuality Vol. 1* examines the blossoming of ideas around sex in Western societies since the eighteenth century.

- The text challenges common ideas about nineteenth-century views of sex and sexuality. Foucault goes on to examine the scientific study of sexuality from the same period, to show how knowledge is constructed, and power can be productive.

- Although Foucault's writing style can make the text difficult to follow, it is helped by the way he frequently anticipates and answers the reader's questions.

Key Themes

Michel Foucault's *The History of Sexuality Vol. 1: The Will to Knowledge* explores how various ideas about sex and new ways of talking about it have developed and spread in modern Western societies since the eighteenth century. The text challenges the "repressive hypothesis,"* which claimed that the dominant classes of society (the wealthy middle classes and the Church) emphasized the reproductive function of sex, while suppressing and silencing its pleasurable qualities. Sex in Western societies came to be restricted and was considered acceptable only in the private space of the married heterosexual* couple's bedroom. According to this premise, even the discussion of sex was suppressed in nineteenth-century society.

Foucault asks important questions—one historical, a second theoretical, and a third historical-political—about the repressive hypothesis. First, he asks whether sexual repression was a historical fact:

> **66** The society that emerged in the nineteenth
> century—bourgeois, capitalist, or industrial society,
> call it what you will—did not confront sex with a
> fundamental refusal of recognition. On the contrary, it
> put into operation an entire machinery for producing
> true discourses concerning it. **99**

Michel Foucault, *The History of Sexuality Vol. 1: The Will to Knowledge*

Did it actually happen? Second, he asks whether power in our society works through repression. Third, he asks whether the concept of sexual liberation is part of the same network of power that it so forcefully denounces, misnaming it as "repression."

Foucault proposes that the call for sexual liberation in the West at the time he was working on the book in fact parallels the history of repression that the liberators wished to oppose. Foucault proposes that, instead of simply repressing sex, the more powerful classes had actually sought to make people talk about it, and to make it an object of scientific analysis. The themes of *Sexuality Vol. 1* are: the relationship between the scientific study of sex and the state's regulation of sexual behavior; the evolution of sex and sexuality as concepts; the role that modern scientific disciplines have played in shaping our understanding of sexuality; and, finally, the relationship between sex, power, and knowledge.

Exploring the Ideas

The most important argument Foucault sets out in *Sexuality Vol. 1* has to do with the relationship between knowledge (in this case, from the study of sexuality), power, and the construction of identity. Foucault challenges the popular view that sexuality has been clearly repressed since the start of bourgeois* society. Instead, he claims that sexuality in the eighteenth and nineteenth centuries became an object of scientific analysis within the budding fields of biology,* demography,* pedagogy,* and psychiatry.* These disciplines produced knowledge about sexual desires, orientations, and preferences that were supposed to be linked to the truth about someone's character. Foucault calls this *scientia sexualis*—the science of sex.

One of the effects of *scientia sexualis*, Foucault argues, is that nineteenth-century society came to view sexuality as deeply connected to a person's identity. In other words, sexuality was viewed as indicating an individual's true self. Scientists began to study people they thought exhibited "abnormal" sexual desires or behavior. The sexuality of the mentally ill, criminals, and sex between people of the same gender whipped up scientists' curiosity. The knowledge scientists gained from their studies led to the creation of distinct categories of individuals based on their sexual preferences.

According to Foucault, the term "homosexual"* was a product of one such study. The term first entered scientific discussion in 1870 through an article by the German neurologist* and psychiatrist Carl Westphal,* who used it to define a particular type of person with a particular kind of character—or as Foucault calls it, "a hermaphrodism* (having both male and female organs) of the soul."[1] Westphal looked at the act of sex between two men and built an entire theory, and identity category, around it. Such categorizations, like *scientia sexualis* as a whole, in turn gave rise to new forms of regulation designed to curb "abnormal" sexual behavior.[2]

Foucault concludes from this that power in the modern period does not operate primarily through direct repression (for instance, stopping people from talking about their sexual fantasies). Instead, power operates through the production of knowledge (gathering detailed information about people's fantasies, and then using that information to develop theories about what makes up normal and abnormal behavior, and laws to uphold those principles). Foucault concludes that a society's knowledge producers (the institutions that analyze human behavior, draw conclusions, and then feed that information back into society) play a central role in influencing its desires and ideals. It is in this sense that Foucault argues power is productive. The idea that our sexual behavior (and for Foucault, our behavior in general) is an effect of the power structures in our societies is among Foucault's most important contributions to the social sciences.*

Language and Expression
The unclear phrasing and complex arguments of *Sexuality Vol. 1* might lead a reader to believe it was aimed at an academic audience, but Foucault intended to intervene in the public debate as much as in academic discussions.

Foucault's efforts to speak to an audience beyond academia can be seen as part of a broader shift in his intellectual thought. For historian François Dosse, the clearest difference between Foucault's work in the 1970s and that of the previous decade is his personal involvement in grassroots activism, especially in the *Groupe d'Information sur les Prisons* (Prison Information Group*), an organization in France fighting for inmates' rights. Dosse argues that the most important "shift in Foucault's position" in the 1970s was to become "personally involved in his theoretical object of study."[3]

This shift, however, is not reflected in Foucault's writing style, which does little to help average readers understand its content. As Foucault himself admitted, his arguments tend to roll out "at the cost of a certain difficulty for the author and the reader."[4] Readers new to Foucault will notice that his work assumes that his audience is familiar with a broad range of cultural phenomena. His arguments are often peppered with hard-to-understand references, while his paragraph-long sentences can make it difficult for even an experienced academic to understand what he is saying. Readers might take comfort, however, in the fact that *Sexuality Vol. 1* is an easy read compared to earlier works of Foucault's, such as *The Birth of the Clinic** (1963) and *The Order of Things** (1966).

Another feature of Foucault's style worth noting is his tendency to advance his arguments by first questioning them. This rhetorical method allows him to construct a text that anticipates and answers the reader's questions—making the work somewhat easier to navigate.

NOTES

1   Michel Foucault, *The History of Sexuality Vol. 1: The Will to Knowledge,* trans. Robert Hurley (London: Penguin Books, 1998), 43.

2   Foucault, *Sexuality Vol. 1,* 45.

3   See Francois Dosse, *History of Structuralism. Volume II. The Sign Sets 1967–Present,* trans. Deborah Glassman (Minneapolis: University of Minnesota Press, 1998), 249.

4   See Paul Rabinow, "Series Preface" in *Michel Foucault: Ethics, Subjectivity and Truth*, ed. Paul Rabinow (New York: The New Press, 1997), vii.

MODULE 6
SECONDARY IDEAS

KEY POINTS

- Foucault's *Sexuality Vol. 1* considers the workings of power, and advances the idea that our very identities are, at least in part, shaped by those who produce knowledge— meaning that even those who resist authority must do so from within the system they are opposing.

- This concept has been questioned and to an extent misunderstood by the academic community, which has led to significant controversies.

- Foucault's fertile work has prompted a huge amount of intellectual debate and academic articles; more recently, the book has been criticized for its failure to consider the role of colonial* oppression and racism in the history he examines ("colonialism" is the policy of settling and exploiting a foreign territory and its people).

Other Ideas

The most important secondary idea in Michel Foucault's *The History of Sexuality Vol. 1: The Will to Knowledge* is his understanding of power as dispersed, or spread out. While his discussion of power might appear secondary, simply supporting his general aim of explaining the constructed nature of sexual categories, it is in fact crucial to understanding the full complexity of his work.

These ideas occupy a central position and are presented clearly in the last chapters, "The Deployment of Sexuality" and "Right of Death and Power over Life." Here, Foucault extends his discussion of sexuality to propose a new theory of power, criticizing the view that power acts in a one-way manner, from top to bottom. Instead, he

> **66** Power comes from below; that is, there is no binary and all-encompassing opposition between rulers and ruled at the root of power relations, and serving as a general matrix. **99**
>
> *The History of Sexuality Vol. 1: The Will to Knowledge*

argues, power is a complex force that enables desires, pleasures, and identities.

Foucault's idea of power as dispersed seeks to explain how power operates and how resistance to power might take place. This proposition was influential in the development both of political activism and of certain principles of post-Marxism* (theoretical approaches grounded in Marxist* theory but extending, reversing, or modifying it) and anarchist* political theory (theory founded on the principle that the institution of hierarchical government is illegitimate). However, Foucault's arguments on power were not without their critics, and the discussions that they set off are instructive.

In the final section, "Right of Death and Power over Life," Foucault reviews the difference between the exercise of power in earlier times and its exercise in modern societies. In earlier times, power acted in a "deductive" way; the ruler would exert his authority by taking his or her subjects' taxes, wealth, land, and life. In modern societies, power is "productive," being used to produce a certain kind of individual through sophisticated methods of regulation and control. Withholding or granting birth control, banning or granting abortion, championing heterosexuality,* and recommending a certain number of children per family are all methods involving the regulation of sexual and reproductive behavior. Modern society uses these means to control the population and ensure citizens follow a certain way of life. In this sense, sex in modern societies is seen as a practice to be administered.

Exploring the Ideas

In *Sexuality Vol. 1* Foucault argues that the ways we think about our sexuality and the sexuality of people around us are closely related to the sexual categories produced by modern scientific institutions. The scientific community has great power over how we perceive human behavior and desire and, in turn, ourselves. When scientists tell us something is unhealthy or unnatural, we believe them. To the extent that we do not question these ideas but take them to be facts, we are already, unknowingly within subject-to-power relations—roughly, the exercise of hierarchical power. Resistance, the effort to rebel against authority, is no different; it takes place within power relations, and cannot be exercised from an external point.

This crucial idea has, however, led to misunderstandings. Foucault has often been misinterpreted as arguing that, since power is everywhere, there is no escape from it and, therefore, resistance is futile.[1] In fact, Foucault argues the opposite. The point of his argument is to challenge the idea that there is one power that we have to oppose. In his words, there is "no binary and all-encompassing opposition between rulers and ruled."[2] Moreover, "Where there is power, there is resistance and yet, or rather consequently, this resistance is never in a position of exteriority in relation to power."[3]

What Foucault meant by this is that any form of resistance has to recognize that it is already involved in power relations. Resistance is not futile; the point is that those who resist must also recognize that they are not doing so from some pure position freed from power. American queer* studies scholar David Halperin* clarifies the kind of power Foucault is talking about, observing that "some of Foucault's critics on the Left may simply have misunderstood his claim, 'power is everywhere' … When he says that 'power is everywhere,' Foucault is not talking about power in the sense of coercive and irresistible force … rather, he is referring to what might be called *liberal* power*—that is, to the kind of power … which takes as its objects 'free subjects' and defines itself wholly in relation to them and to their freedom."[4]

Institutions, in other words, have exerted authority by regulating how sex is talked about, and what sexual behaviors or preferences a society deems "healthy" or "unhealthy." These social codes have, in turn, gained a life of their own (so to speak), shaping views and behaviors in ways rulers could not have foreseen. Power and sexuality are linked in modernity* because, in this era, sexuality is regulated both directly (through rules) and indirectly (through social codes that cannot be said to come from any one specific source).

Overlooked

Sexuality Vol. 1 has provoked a rich intellectual debate, and has been followed by a considerable number of academic texts discussing the various points it raises. Scholars have questioned some of the work's ideas, including the text's Eurocentrism*—that is, the extent to which its arguments are limited to European culture, and neglect to consider the sexuality or viewpoint of other races and ethnic groups (including people who still lived under European colonial rule, or were just gaining independence, at the time Foucault was writing).

In 1988, only 12 years after the book's original publication, the Eurocentricity of Foucault's thought became the subject of debate. In *The Predicament of Culture* (1988), the American anthropologist James Clifford* warned that the "scrupulously ethnocentric" nature of Foucault's approach "has avoided all comparative appeals to other worlds of meaning."[5] Similar objections have come from the field of postcolonial* studies (inquiry into the various cultural and social legacies of colonialism). The scholar Gayatri Chakravorty Spivak,* for example, in her famous essay "Can the Subaltern Speak?", positioned Foucault within a Western literary tradition that denies voice and agency (the power to act) to non-Western populations.

It was not until 1995, with the US anthropologist* Ann Stoler's*

Race and the Education of Desire: Foucault's History of Sexuality and the Colonial Order of Things (1995), that a fertile discussion and radical rereading of Foucault from a postcolonial angle truly began. Stoler argued that Foucault ignores how Western modernity was shaped to a large extent through its interaction with non-European populations and, more importantly, through racism, colonialism and slavery. While sympathetic to Foucault's ideas, Stoler maintained that Foucault presents a history of European sexuality that fails to see the ways that European middle-class identity was largely formed in opposition to colonized cultures. "Why for Foucault," she asked forcefully, "do colonial bodies never figure as a possible site of the articulation of nineteenth-century European sexuality?"[6]

By rethinking the history of sexuality based on the unequal power between European colonizers and the colonized (in Africa, Asia, and Oceania), the book brought to light a largely neglected side of Foucault's text: that of race in relation to the way bourgeois* people grew to see themselves. Without abandoning Foucault's overall aim of disturbing stereotypical ideas of sexual identities, Stoler's text offered a productive, culturally specific critique of *Sexuality Vol. 1*, and opened up new ways of using Foucault's ideas in the study of colonial rule.[7]

NOTES

1   David Halperin, *Saint Foucault: Towards a Gay Hagiography* (New York: Oxford University Press, 1995), 18.

2   Michel Foucault, *The History of Sexuality Vol. 1: The Will to Knowledge,* trans. Robert Hurley (London: Penguin Books, 1998), 94.

3   Foucault, *Sexuality Vol. 1*, 95.

4   Halperin, *Saint Foucault*, 18.

5   James Clifford, *The Predicament of Culture: Twentieth-Century Ethnography, Literature, and Art* (Cambridge, Mass: Harvard University Press, 1988), 264–5.

6   See Ann Laura Stoler, *Race and the Education of Desire: Foucault's History of Sexuality and the Colonial Order of Things* (Durham, North Carolina: Duke University Press, 1995), i.

7   Stoler, *Race and the Education of Desire*, 1–2.

MODULE 7
ACHIEVEMENT

KEY POINTS

- Foucault's novel approach introduced a new way of thinking about sexuality, the production of knowledge, and the workings of power that have since influenced various fields across the humanities* and social sciences.*

- The first publication of *Sexuality Vol. 1* in 1976, and its 1978 English translation, had a great impact on homosexual* and queer* activists—activists who wish to challenge widely held assumptions regarding sexuality and gender* identity with the aim of reshaping structures of power and the balance of equality.

- Although recognized as a groundbreaking work, the book has also been criticized by feminist* and postcolonial* scholars who viewed it as androcentric* (focusing on the male experience) and Eurocentric.*

Assessing the Argument

Michel Foucault's *The History of Sexuality Vol. 1: The Will to Knowledge* is highly original in the way it opposes the Freudo-Marxist* analysis of sexuality then dominant in intellectual circles. Instead, Foucault proposes that sex is a set of ideas constructed by society and shaped in and by scientific institutions, and that these ideas are used to regulate individuals and populations. Foucault makes this argument through a complex historical and theoretical analysis that traces the rise, at the end of the seventeenth century, of a new discipline that viewed sex as an object of scientific study. This new approach informed the way people were labeled as normal or abnormal.

Foucault's approach gave birth to a whole genre of studies around

> **❝** Pleasure and power do not cancel or turn back against one another; they seek out, overlap, and reinforce one another. They are linked together by complex mechanisms and devices of excitation and excitement. **❞**
>
> Michel Foucault, *The History of Sexuality Vol 1: The Will to Knowledge*

sexuality. These studies, which expanded substantially during the 1990s and now hold a leading place in scholarly debates, regard sexuality as an effect of power and not necessarily in strict opposition to it.

This latter point relates to another original idea that set the text apart from similar studies: Foucault's understanding of power. He made the significant claim that power does not only work in negative ways—it does not, for example, serve simply to prohibit or repress instinctual drives (such as the "sex drive") that desire unimpeded expression. Nor does power work only in a simple top-down direction. For Foucault, power is also productive in the sense that it creates preferences, orientations, and desires in people.

This idea of power not as a total force but, rather, as a set of relations proved key for the development of post-Marxist* political theory. Foucault's work has been central for post-Marxists, such as the Argentinian political-theorist Ernesto Laclau,* the Belgian political-theorist Chantal Mouffe,* and the Italian philosopher Antonio Negri.*

Achievement in Context

Although the title of Foucault's work indicates that it is a history of sexuality, it would be simplistic to see it only as a historical text in the conventional sense. Foucault never thought of himself as a professional historian; instead he sought to expose the basic assumptions in our understanding of modern Western societies. As such, the work must also be seen as an examination of how concepts such as truth, knowledge, and power relate to the way sexual practices are represented and understood.

By challenging these positions, Foucault's work offered new ways of thinking about sexuality—seeing it as an effect of social conditions and not as pure instinct. Furthermore, Foucault's idea of "power" as multiple arrangements of relations and forces, and not just the use or threat of force by a ruler, has had a long-lasting influence in the intellectual world.

Foucault's text was also groundbreaking outside of academia. Following first publication in 1976 and its English translation two years later, the book had a significant impact on gay and queer activists during the 1980s and 1990s. Professor David Halperin, a scholar noted for his contribution to queer theory, has observed that when gay activists in New York during the late 1980s were asked about their influences, they would give "without the slightest hesitation or a single exception, the following answer: Michel Foucault, *The History of Sexuality Volume I*."[1]

Limitations

Although the claims that Foucault makes are truly pioneering, due to the book's short length they are not always analyzed in depth. In this sense, the text as a whole seems to be a promise of something more that will follow. This makes sense as *Sexuality Vol. 1* was intended to be the first of a six-volume work. It is also worth noting that the text is not as thorough and rigorous as one might expect to find in a historical study—a point that has been seen as a serious weakness.[2]

Among the book's most frequently cited limitations is that it focuses almost exclusively on the role of sexuality in Western modernity.* One might counter this claim, however, by arguing that the object of Foucault's study, "modernity,"* refers not only to a historical period of the Western world, but to a set of practices, approaches to knowledge, and institutions that have spread globally. For example, the discussion of sexuality based on scientific knowledge that has (now, or in the past) labeled certain practices as "perversions" or "pathological" has by now extended to other parts of the world. *Sexuality Vol. 1,* in other words, arrives at conclusions that can be analyzed in relation to non-European societies and populations.

Other criticisms of the text are harder to dismiss. For instance, Foucault's only mention of sexuality in civilizations other than in current, or ancient, Europe occurs in Part Three, "Scientia Sexualis,"* where he contrasts what he calls the "two great procedures for producing the truth of sex."[3] Here he argues that in China, Japan, India, Rome, and the Arab-Muslim world truth about sex has been understood by means of *ars erotica,** that is to say from teachings about pleasure and experience itself. This is in contrast to modern Western societies, where truth about sex is informed by scientia sexualis, a means of understanding sexuality based on the production of knowledge about it, such as scientific study or the ritual of confession.* This analysis has sparked criticism from scholars such as the Tunisian sociologist Fathi Triki,* who has termed it both naïve and inaccurate.[4]

Sexuality Vol. 1 has also been criticized by feminist critics for its "blindness to sexual violence"[5] and for being androcentric—that is, for focusing on the experience of men.[6] The most frequently censured part of the text is Foucault's account of a case in 1867, when a farmer from the town of Lapcourt, France, was turned over to the authorities for having "obtained a few caresses from a little girl."[7] For Foucault the remarkable thing in the story is that, as a result of his act, the man became the object of "a judicial action, a medical intervention, a careful clinical examination, and an entire theoretical elaboration."[8] For Foucault, the way the man was turned into a "pure object of medicine and knowledge"[9] indicates how, through the use of legal-psychiatric categories, sexual acts in modern times came to be seen as revealing a person's inner self (in this case, a man capable of sexual harassment or rape). Feminist writers have criticized this interpretation for ignoring the victim and the violence she suffered, and focusing only on the point of view of the man accused of committing the act.[10]

NOTES

1   See David Halperin, *Saint Foucault: Towards a Gay Hagiography* (New York: Oxford University Press, 1995), 16.

2   See, for example, Jeremy R. Carrette, *Foucault and Religion: Spiritual Corporality and Political Spirituality* (London: Routledge, 2000), 131; Elizabeth A. Clark, "Foucault, The Fathers and Sex," *Journal of the American Academy of Religion* 56, no .4 (1988): 625.

3   Michel Foucault, *The History of Sexuality Vol. 1: The Will to Knowledge,* trans. Robert Hurley (London: Penguin Books, 1998), 57.

4   Janet Afary and Kevin B. Anderson, "Foucault, Gender and Male Homosexualities in Mediterranean and Muslim Society," in *Foucault and the Iranian Revolution: Gender and the Seductions of Islamism* (Chicago: University of Chicago Press, 2005), 138–62, citation on 141.

5   Kelly H. Ball, "'More or Less Raped': Foucault, Causality, and Feminist Critiques of Sexual Violence," *philoSOPHIA* 3, no.1 (2013): 53.

6   Kate Soper, "Productive Contradictions," in *Up Against Foucault: Explorations of Some Tensions Between Foucault and Feminism*, ed. Caroline Ramazanoglu (New York: Routledge), 29.

7   Foucault, *Sexuality Vol. 1*, 31.

8   Foucault, *Sexuality Vol. 1*, 31.

9   Foucault, *Sexuality Vol. 1*, 31.

10 For a discussion see Ball, "'More or Less Raped'."

MODULE 8
PLACE IN THE AUTHOR'S WORK

KEY POINTS

- Published in 1976, *Sexuality Vol. 1* is among Foucault's last works, and marks an important moment in the evolution of his thought.

- As with Foucault's other books, *Sexuality Vol. 1* is concerned with power and knowledge and the construction of identity, but it approaches these in a new way, through the concepts of "governmentality"* (practices of governing that aim to shape citizens' conduct instead of openly suppressing them) and "biopower"* (a term Foucault uses for an "explosion" of techniques used to subjugate individual bodies and entire populations).

- Foucault's influence on the development of the fields of queer* theory and gender* and sexuality* studies is undisputed; together with his *Discipline and Punish,* * the three volumes of *The History of Sexuality* are his most well-known and most frequently cited books.

Positioning

Michel Foucault's *The History of Sexuality Vol. 1: The Will to Knowledge* examines the subject of sexuality. His views on the workings of power can be traced to earlier texts. The most obvious is Discipline and Punish, dealing with prisons, which he published a year earlier, in 1975. Foucault regarded *Sexuality Vol. 1* as a continuation of this earlier book.[1]

In *Discipline and Punish*, Foucault discussed changes in the Western penal system (especially prisons) during the eighteenth and nineteenth centuries. He argued persuasively that, around that time, the physical abuse of offenders gradually gave way to punishment based on

> ❝ The omnipresence of power: not because it has the privilege of consolidating everything under its invincible unity, but because it is produced from one moment to the next, at every point, or rather in every relation from one point to another. Power is everywhere; not because it embraces everything, but because it comes from everywhere. ❞
>
> Michel Foucault, *The History of Sexuality Vol. 1: The Will to Knowledge*

analyzing the criminal for reasons why he or she committed offences, and advancing scientific research into the so-called "criminal mind." Such research was also used to determine whether the criminal could be reformed, made "normal," and reintegrated into society. Rather than sentencing an offender to death, doctors would seek to eradicate the bad behavior. During that time, "a corpus [body] of knowledge, techniques, 'scientific' discourses is formed and becomes entangled with the practice of the power to punish."[2] Traces of these ideas are evident in *Sexuality Vol.* 1, which is also concerned with how knowledge is used to produce new forms of regulation and control.

According to scholars such as Alan D. Schrift,* Foucault's writing career can be divided into three separate periods: an earlier "archaeological" phase, during which he was focused on questions of discourse and language ("archaeology" is the study of history through the physical remains of human activity and the analysis of objects); a second "genealogical"* phase focusing on the relation between power and knowledge; and a third "ethical" phase concerned with subjectivity* (here meaning the ways in which individual selfhood, or identity, develops).

For Schrift, the archaeological period included *Madness and Civilization** (1964), *The Order of Things** (1966), and *The Archaeology of Knowledge** (1969), which share a concern with "the relations of knowledge, language, truth." The genealogical period, which focuses specifically on power, includes *Discipline and Punish* (1975) and *The History of Sexuality Vol. 1* (1976). The ethical period includes *The History of Sexuality Vols. 2** and *3** (1984), which stand out from Foucault's previous works in their focus on the "construction of the ethical/sexual subject or self."[3] However, these categories are in no way final, and they have often been contested as overly simplistic. Foucault himself would likely have resisted such labeling since he was skeptical about fixed categories, and because of his fascination with the motives of scholars when they insisted on making them.

Integration

Among the most important of Foucault's ideas appears in a complex discussion he sets out halfway through *Sexuality Vol. 1*, regarding the ways power operates in modern societies.

According to Foucault, power—and, specifically, *modern* power—does not operate from top to bottom, as "there is no binary and all-encompassing opposition between rulers and ruled."[4] As such, there is no single and totalitarian "power" that represses and prohibits desires: there are power relations that are aided and strengthened by different techniques that aim to control, as he describes it, "men's existence, men as living bodies."[5]

Foucault introduces the term "biopower" to refer to this idea, which is one of the most important concepts in his later work. In particular, biopower relates to another concept of Foucault: "governmentality." He coined this term to define practices of governing that aim to shape citizens' conduct (their behavior as well as their thoughts), instead of openly suppressing them—for instance, the use of scientific knowledge about sex to regulate it.

Although Foucault's individual texts share many themes, they also express quite noticeable differences that reflect the evolution of his thinking. For instance, Foucault's early works, such as *Madness and*

Civilization and *The Birth of the Clinic** (1963) were influenced by structuralist* thought, in contrast to his later works, which could be termed poststructuralist.*

Structuralism is a theoretical approach, according to which elements of culture become intelligible if studied in relation to the larger structures and systems in which they belong. Poststructuralism questions the existence of these structures—and, indeed, the belief that we can be entirely certain that objective knowledge is possible at all, given that it is impossible to escape the cultural assumptions with which we begin any analysis.

In *The Archaeology of Knowledge*, Foucault describes his early works as a "very imperfect sketch,"[6] finding it "mortifying … that [his] analyses were conducted in terms of cultural totality."[7] This quote illustrates the difference not only between Foucault's early and late works, but the difference between structuralism and poststructuralism.

Structuralist thought seeks to understand a particular element of culture through the society's structures of which it is a part. So, for instance, in *The Birth of the Clinic* Foucault traces the development of the medical profession as a whole through a history of the medical clinic, in order to consider how knowledge of the human body and human health is produced by what he calls the "medical gaze."* A poststructuralist, by contrast, would not claim to be able to understand the subject in its entirety, admitting instead that, as a participant in the study, he or she could not help but be biased. In other words, in his later writings Foucault is aware that he himself is writing from within an institution, as a professor in twentieth-century France, and that this limits the scope of what he can understand.

Significance

Although scholarly discussions of sexuality have shifted since the book was written, *Sexuality Vol. 1* remains one of the key and most quoted texts in the fields of queer theory and gender and sexuality studies.

Queer theory is an approach to cultural analysis that begins by acknowledging the instability and uncertainty of sexual identity and of knowledge itself; sexuality studies is inquiry into the ways in which sexuality (roughly, our preferences and orientations) is constructed and understood.

Since it was first published, the theory that Foucault proposed in *Sexuality Vol. 1* has regularly been cited and treated as a point of reference by highly respected scholars across the world. According to the *Times Higher Education magazine*, Foucault was the most quoted author in the humanities* and social sciences* in 2007.[8]

Sexuality Vol. 1 can be seen to bring together and extend parts of Foucault's earlier thought. The text develops and voices more fully the relationship between power, knowledge, and the body that is central to all his work. If one were to state the aim of Foucault's academic career, it would perhaps be: to understand how power operates across societies and academic disciplines, to understand the relationship between power and knowledge, and to understand how the human body, human sexuality, and concepts such as madness, criminality, and surveillance have historically been used to observe citizens' behavior or alter it. *Sexuality Vol. 1* is an important step toward his goal.

NOTES

1   See David Macey, *The Lives of Michel Foucault* (New York: Pantheon, 1993), 354.

2   Michel Foucault, *Discipline and Punish*, trans. Alan Sheridan (New York: Random House, 1977), 23.

3   See Alan D. Schrift, *Nietzsche's French Legacy: A Genealogy of Poststructuralism* (London: Routledge, 1995), 35–7.

4   Michel Foucault, *The History of Sexuality Vol. 1: The Will to Knowledge,* trans. Robert Hurley (London: Penguin Books, 1998), 98.

5   Foucault, *Sexuality Vol. 1,* 89.

6   Michel Foucault, *The Archaeology of Knowledge,* trans. A. M. Sheridan Smith (London: Tavistock Publications Limited, 1972), 15.

7   Foucault, *Archaeology of Knowledge*, 15.

8   "Most Cited Authors of Books in the Humanities, 2007," *Times Higher Education*, accessed November 15, 2015, http://www.timeshighereducation. co.uk/405956.article.

SECTION 3
IMPACT

MODULE 9
THE FIRST RESPONSES

KEY POINTS

- *The History of Sexuality Vol. 1* was received negatively by many scholars on publication; feminist critics debated about the book intensely, some welcoming Michel Foucault's questioning of sexual categories, others criticizing some of his views on sexual violence.

- While Foucault responded to a few of his critics in interviews, for the most part he did not engage with the debate.

- The shift in focus in the second and third volumes of *History of Sexuality* can however be interpreted as an effort on Foucault's part to take his critics' points on board.

Criticism

When it was first published, Michel Foucault's *The History of Sexuality Vol. 1: The Will to Knowledge* received a great deal of unfavorable attention.[1] In its first years the most serious criticism focused on particular aspects of the text rather than on the work as whole. While a lot of criticism came from a Marxist* and psychoanalytic* point of view, perhaps the most lasting and fertile early discussions of *Sexuality Vol. 1* emerged from a feminist* background.

The American academic and writer Biddy Martin* warned in 1982 of "the danger that Foucault's challenges to traditional categories, if taken to a 'logical' conclusion … could make the question of women's oppression obsolete."[2] She further warned feminists "not [to] be seduced by the work of Foucault."[3] Although feminists were for the most part sympathetic to Foucault's method as well as to his belief in the constructed nature of sexual categories, writers like Martin

> ❝ The essential point is that sex was not only a matter of sensation and pleasure, of law and taboo, but also of truth and falsehood, that the truth of sex became something fundamental, useful, or dangerous, precious or formidable: in short, that sex was constituted as a problem of truth. ❞
>
> Michel Foucault, *The History of Sexuality Vol. 1: The Will to Knowledge*

pointed out the limitations of Foucault's work when it came to addressing their social demands toward equality between the sexes.

Other feminists criticized Foucault's ideas about sexual violence. The first article to raise the issue was "Our Costs and Their Benefits" (1978) by the French feminist scholar and activist Monique Plaza.* The article addressed Foucault's views on France's rape law that he voiced in 1977, a year after the publication of *Sexuality Vol. 1*, during a debate over amending the law. Extending some of the claims he made in *Sexuality Vol. 1*, Foucault claimed that cases of rape should be seen and punished by the law in the same way as all other acts of "violence"—a punch in the face, for example.[4] He argued that the attacker's "sexuality" should not be punished by the law.

Plaza's article, in which she accused Foucault of "de-sexualizing rape," looked to take apart Foucault's argument. According to Plaza, Foucault saw sexuality as an effect of a deployment (that is, the use) of power, of which women's bodies were the prime victims. Plaza claimed that by "not forbidding the deployment of power which has as its object of privileged appropriation the bodies of women"[5] (that is to say, by not forbidding the use of force to take control of women's bodies), Foucault ends up reproducing the same power structures that he almost certainly opposed (in this case, the ways in which men have historically taken possession of female bodies). As *two British commentators have written*, "in seeking to rewrite the law on rape in such a way as to punish violence but decriminalise sexuality, he is defending men's existing right to possess women's bodies."[6]

Responses

Because Foucault died in 1984, eight years after *Sexuality Vol. 1* was originally published in France and six years after its English translation, and most of the scholarly critiques on Foucault's work were written in the 1980s and 1990s, he did not have a chance to reply to most of them.

We have some responses to his first critics, however. In an interview a few years after the publication of Sexuality Vol. 1, Foucault responded to the feminist criticism that he had dismissed sexual violence and desexualized rape.[7] He stated: "I say 'freedom of sexual choice' and not 'freedom of sexual acts' because there are sexual acts like rape which should not be permitted."[8]

One of the most common accusations against Foucault is that, since he sees power as not being exclusively localized in government and the state but as exercised throughout the social body (the whole of society), resistance is impossible. However, in a later interview, he directly rejected this accusation, stating that "the claim that 'you see power everywhere, thus there is no room for freedom' seems to me absolutely inadequate. The idea that power is a system of domination that controls everything and leaves no room for freedom cannot be attributed to me."[9]

Conflict and Consensus

Foucault saw his work as necessarily subject to change, and although his books share many of the same themes, the differences between his earliest studies and his last show the extent to which he sought to develop and refine his ideas.

There is also evidence that some of the changes in his methodology and approach were as a result of criticisms of his earlier work. For instance, one might interpret his focus, in *Vol. 2** and *Vol. 3** of *The History of Sexuality*, on practices of resistance against certain social systems of power as a response to critics' claims that *Vol. 1* failed to fully address these. Foucault himself never directly commented on this—but the shift in tone between *Vol. 1* and the following two volumes is significant, and could well have been influenced by the criticism of the first volume. This shift also resulted in a far more sympathetic response from feminist critics to Foucault's later work on the "care of the self" in *Vol. 3*. For many, its discussion of the nature of sexual identity and its understanding of sexual behavior had an ethical dimension; the text offered a model for understanding individual identity in terms of our responsibilities to others.[10]

Finally, it is worth noting that for all the negative criticism it received at first, Foucault's *Sexuality Vol. 1* brought about a new understanding of how sexuality, desire, and institutional power relate to each other. While some of his ideas on specific issues such as rape remain controversial, his main ideas regarding the relationship between knowledge, power, and identity remain highly influential. Foucault himself continues to be among the most cited authors in the humanities* and social sciences,* and one of the most influential scholars since the 1970s.

NOTES

1   Daniel Defert, "Chronology," in *A Companion to Foucault*, eds. Christopher Falzon et al. (Chichester: Wiley & Sons, 2013), 63.

2   Biddy Martin, "Feminism, Criticism, and Foucault," *New German Critique* 27 (1982): 17.

3   Martin, "Feminism, Criticism, and Foucault," 7.

4   Michel Foucault, "La Folie Encircle," cited in Dani Cavallaro, *French Feminist Theory: An Introduction* (London: Continuum, 2003), 102.

5   See Monique Plaza, "Our Costs and Their Benefits," in *Sex in Question: French Materialist Feminism*, eds. Diana Leonard and Lisa Adkins (London: Taylor & Francis, 1996), 185.

6   See Diana Leonard and Lisa Adkins, "Reconstructing French Feminism: Commodification, Materialism and Sex," in *Sex in Question*, 18.

7   See Monique Plaza, "Our Costs and Their Benefits," in *Sex in Question*, 185.

8   Michel Foucault, "Sexual Choice, Sexual Act," trans. James O'Higgins, in *Michel Foucault: Ethics, Subjectivity and Truth*, ed. Paul Rabinow (New York: The New Press, 1997), 143.

9   Michel Foucault, "The Ethics of the Concern for Self as a Practice of Freedom," trans. P. Aranaov and D. McGrawth, in *Michel Foucault: Ethics, Subjectivity and Truth*, ed. Paul Rabinow (New York: The New Press, 1997), 293.

10   See Ladelle McWhorter, *Bodies and Pleasures: Foucault and the Politics of Sexual Normalization* (Bloomington: Indiana University Press, 1999), 196; and Amy Allen, "Foucault, Feminism and the Self: The Politics of Personal Transformation," *Feminism and the Final Foucault*, eds. Dianna Taylor and Karen Vintges (Chicago: University of Illinois Press, 2004), 235–57.

MODULE 10
THE EVOLVING DEBATE

KEY POINTS

- Foucault's *Sexuality Vol. 1* has changed the way scholars think about sexuality, and influenced the development of new academic fields, including queer* theory and gender* and sexuality* studies.

- Foucault's ideas on power are, however, at odds with certain schools of thought—most notably, orthodox Marxism,* psychoanalysis,* and some branches of feminist* criticism, each of which is based on an idea of centralized power.

- Most recently, Foucault's concepts of biopower* and governmentality* have inspired the field of governmentality studies,* which uses his ideas to examine how liberal* societies are governed.

Uses and Problems

The History of Sexuality Vol. 1: The Will to Knowledge is one of Michel Foucault's most quoted and influential texts, and has had a considerable impact on the work of important thinkers and even whole intellectual schools. The scholars who are deeply engaged with the text are numerous and their activity ranges over diverse fields, from cultural studies* (a discipline proposing an anthropological* reading of social relations) and philosophy, to literature and anthropology.

However, the ideas Foucault advances in *Sexuality Vol. 1* are also at odds with certain schools of thought that take issue with Foucault's theory of power being dispersed (spread out). This argument conflicts with disciplines such as feminism, orthodox Marxism, and psychoanalysis, each of which is informed by a more centralized

> **❝**Until Freud at least, the discourse on sex—the discourse of scholars and theoreticians—never ceased to hide the thing it was speaking about. We could take all these things that were said, the painstaking precautions and analyses, as so many procedures meant to evade the unbearable, too hazardous, truth of sex.**❞**
>
> Michel Foucault, *The History of Sexuality Vol. 1: The Will to Knowledge*

conception of power. Feminists see power in relation to male domination and a society's patriarchal* (male-ruled) views. For orthodox Marxists, power is concentrated in the hands of those with money and social status. For psychoanalysts, power shows itself in concepts such as the Law of the Father* (a term used by the French psychoanalyst Jacques Lacan* to describe the law prohibiting taboo actions such as incest). Each of these approaches is at odds with Foucault's views.

Feminist critics in particular, whose focus is closest to the subject matter of *Sexuality Vol. 1*, underline how Foucault's ideas are not suited for expressing resistance against patriarchy and male domination. Further, they point to the way Foucault is unclear in positions toward themes such as rape and sexual violence.

Schools of Thought

Sexuality Vol. 1 does not belong to any one discipline. The text has fueled broad intellectual debate across the humanities* and social sciences* and radically changed the course of academic work on sexuality, power, and knowledge.

Scholars of queer theory and gender and sexuality studies have drawn from Foucault's ideas to question the standard sexual categories such as man/woman, and homosexual*/heterosexual.* Instead, they regard sexuality as "a historically singular experience"—something that changes and evolves depending on the historical period.[1] As the cultural historian Tamsin Spargo* argues in *Queer Studies and Foucault,* Foucault "can be seen as a catalyst [and] a point of departure" for queer theory, "an example and antecedent but also as a continuing irritant, a bit of grit that is still provoking the production of new ideas."[2] The American queer studies scholar David Halperin* likewise notes that, since the publication in English of *Sexuality Vol. 1* in 1978, progress in the field of sexuality studies "has been rapid and scholarly activity has been intense."[3]

Foucault's focus on the body is particularly useful here, as his move away from understanding individuals as stable beings with a given identity was a useful springboard for further study. It helped scholars who were trying to formulate a theory of sexual or gender oppression without accepting the idea that gender or sexual differences are fixed, natural identities.

Foucault's approach was of notable assistance to thinkers such as the US gender scholar Judith Butler* and Eve Sedgwick,* the authors of *Gender Trouble* (1990) and *Epistemology* of the Closet* (1990) respectively—among the first texts to introduce Foucault's *Sexuality Vol. 1* to university humanities departments, especially in the United States. Following Foucault's approach, both works attempt to challenge standard understandings of sexual categories (in Butler's case, male/ female; in Sedgwick's case, gay/straight). It is partly thanks to these books that Foucault is regarded as an intellectual father of queer theory and of gender and sexuality studies.

David Halperin has also helped popularize Foucault's ideas in academia. Among other titles, he wrote *One Hundred Years of Homosexuality and Other Essays on Greek Love* (1990), in which he employs a framework inspired by Foucault to examine the practices and values around sex between men in ancient Greece in contrast to those of bourgeois* (that is, modern Western) societies. With this book, and his biography *Saint Foucault: Toward a Gay Hagiography*

(1995), Halperin has contributed to the spread of Foucault's ideas in the humanities.

In Current Scholarship

The ideas Foucault advanced in *Sexuality Vol. 1* have not only influenced academic debates about sexuality. Since the early 1990s, Foucault's ideas have been applied across the humanities and social sciences—and, most recently, in debates about governance.

Particularly noteworthy is Foucault's influence on the field known as governmentality studies—a term derived from Foucault's concept of governmentality that he developed in the last years of his life to describe the way power (which "governs") shapes subjects, or individuals, including their thoughts and beliefs ("mentality"). Although Foucault coined this term some years after the book's publication, *Sexuality Vol. 1* first advanced the ideas of dispersed power on which it is based. Foucault termed this power "biopower"*—that is to say, a power coming from "innumerable points, in the interplay of non-egalitarian [that is, unequal] and mobile [that is, changeable] relations" that seeks to regulate life.[4]

Governmentality studies, which is based on the work of a number of theorists, including the leading British sociologist Nikolas Rose,* borrows directly from Foucault's ideas. The field focuses on the ways that governance is exercised in liberal* societies ("liberal" is here used in the economic sense, describing the social consequence of the system of capitalism*). According to this school, power in liberal societies is not merely repressive and prohibiting but is distributed across institutions and mechanisms and uses techniques of governance that attempt to shape the conduct of the population. This idea draws directly from Foucault's understanding of how knowledge is produced, and from his claim that turning sex into an object of scientific analysis and using the findings from that research to categorize pathologies (illnesses) and perversions, finally led to new ways for the state to control its citizens.

Academic writing on governmentality in these fields has, in turn, led to renewed interest, since the early 2000s, on the relationship between power and the economy—and particularly on the economic doctrine of neoliberalism,*[5] according to which, government interference in the workings of the market and the national economy is to be discouraged, whatever the social consequences.

NOTES

1 See Michel Foucault, , trans. Robert Hurley (New York: Random House, 2012), 4.

2 Tamsin Spargo, (Cambridge: Icon books, 1999), 17; David Halperin, (New York: Oxford University Press, 1995), 10.

3 David Halperin, *One Hundred Years of Homosexuality: And Other Essays on Greek Love* (London: Routledge, 1990), 34.

4 Michel Foucault, trans. Robert Hurley(London: Penguin Books, 1998), 94.

5 See Wendy Larner, "Neo-liberalism: Policy, Ideology, Governmentality," 63 (2000): 5–25; Nancy Fraser, "From Discipline to Flexibilization? Rereading Foucault in the Shadow of Globalization," 10, no. 2 (2003): 160–71.

MODULE 11
IMPACT AND INFLUENCE TODAY

KEY POINTS

- Foucault's *Sexuality Vol. 1* is a highly respected and widely cited text that has directly shaped academic debates around sexuality, and indirectly influenced the public understanding of gender* and sexual orientation.*

- Foucault's work is often cited as a prime example of poststructuralist* thought for its skepticism toward universal truths; this, however, puts it at odds with liberalism.*

- The controversy surrounding some of Foucault's ideas regarding sexuality, the binary models of man/woman or straight/gay, and the constructed nature of all knowledge are also what make his work a continuing source of interest.

Position

Michel Foucault's *The History of Sexuality Vol. 1: The Will to Knowledge* is considered a groundbreaking text across the humanities* and social sciences.* The work has been widely cited, and both its main and secondary ideas have been widely used across disciplines in the French- and English-speaking academic world. For instance, academic journals such as the *Journal of the History of Sexuality and Sexualities*, founded in 1990 and 1998 respectively, are heavily indebted to Foucault's method, scope, and approach. In addition, Foucault's ideas have shaped discussions about sexualities within gay, lesbian, and feminist communities, as well as in activist language and practice. The queer* theorist David Halperin* further notes that the politics of HIV* activists in the 1980s were strongly informed by *Sexuality Vol. 1*.[1]

❝ We must ... abandon the hypothesis that modern industrial societies ushered in an age of increased sexual repression. We have not only witnessed a visible explosion of unorthodox sexualities; but—and this is the important point—a deployment quite different from the law, even if it is locally dependent on procedures of prohibition, has ensured ... the proliferation of specific pleasures and the multiplication of disparate sexualities. It has been said that ... the agencies of power [have] taken such care to feign ignorance of the thing they prohibited ... But ... the opposite ... has become apparent. **❞**

Michel Foucault, *The History of Sexuality Vol. 1: The Will to Knowledge*

While Foucault's line of reasoning in *Sexuality Vol. 1* is not widely known among the general public, for those familiar with his thought, his influence is clear in today's public debates about sexual minorities. In particular, Foucault's argument that sexuality is a product of social and historical circumstances, and not merely biologically determined, has greatly—if indirectly—influenced popular debates about gender identity* and sexual orientation. Moreover, the idea, largely associated with Foucault, that sexuality is used by institutions to control and make productive the lives of the population (for example, by championing reproduction and the nuclear family), has been highly influential within contemporary artistic production, such as in the work of the New York-based artist David Wojnarowicz.*[2]

Wojnarowicz was a prominent AIDS activist in the 1980s and 1990s. In his memoirs of this period chronicling his activism, Wojnarowicz wrote at length about his disgust with the marginalization and stigmatization of AIDS victims, particularly gay men, who were branded as a "risk" group. He built on Foucault's ideas about the way sexuality is used to diagnose people as "immoral" or "diseased," documenting the way AIDS was employed by politicians to justify demonizing homosexuals.*

Foucault's work has also been itself the subject of artistic production, for example the 1993 BBC documentary *Michel Foucault: Beyond Good and Evil* that offers a portrait of Foucault's life and work,[3] or the acclaimed art installation 24h Foucault by the Swiss artist Thomas Hirschhorn.*[4]

The book's relevance extends beyond its immediate subject matter. This is the case in particular for the arguments Foucault put forward in the last two parts of *Sexuality Vol. 1*: part 4 "The Deployment of Sexuality" and part 5 "Right of Death and Power over Life," where he analyzed the idea of power in modern societies. This has influenced debates in the medical sciences, such as clinical psychiatry,* regarding the way health care is linked to society's systems of social control.[5]

Interaction

Among the schools of thought most skeptical about Foucault's work is that of liberalism; social liberals are concerned with the progression of civil rights, democracy, and social equality. Liberal approaches value factors such as rationality, choice, autonomy (the ability to act without coercion), and equal rights. Liberal feminists,* for instance, insist that women and men should be given the same opportunities in society, believing that promoting women's social inclusion (including in the work place) will advance gender equality. This view assumes certain universal truths, for example that men and women are equal, and that all human beings deserve basic rights. It is incompatible with poststructuralism (including Foucault's approach—*Sexuality Vol. 1* is often taken to be a good example of poststructuralist thought), which mistrusts universal, humanist values and contends that all so-called "truths" are in fact dependent on other factors.

For the same reason, liberal feminists have often criticized Foucault and his followers for supposedly not having anything in their theoretical approach that would support women's struggles against gender inequality and patriarchy.* Foucault claims that the way we understand gender categories is the product of a social construct and not derived from the actual biological differences between the two genders. This challenges the liberal belief in the existence of two naturally separate and opposed sexes, male and female.

Liberal feminists also criticize Foucault's anti–essentialist* ideas (that is, his belief that there are no deep, real differences, such as male/female or straight/gay). For example, the American law and philosophy professor Martha Nussbaum,* in her 1999 article "The Professor of Parody: The Hip Defeatism of Judith Butler,*" forcefully attacked the tendency in feminist thought to follow Foucault. Nussbaum critiques the feminist theorist Judith Butler who, she argues, "seems to many young scholars to define what feminism is now."[6] She also attacks Foucault for not being able to come up with a concept of resistance against oppression. Nussbaum argues that Foucault's approaches to sexuality lack "a normative theory of social justice and human dignity"[7] leading to "quietism [calm acceptance] and retreat."[8]

The Continuing Debate

Foucault's contribution stands as a lasting challenge to all theoretical traditions that treat sexual behavior as something biologically determined. More particularly, *Sexuality Vol. 1* confronts positivist* disciplines such as biology or, for that matter, biological anthropology* ("positivist" here refers to the position that knowledge derives from observation; "biological anthropology" is a field that concerns the study of human behavior in the light of our deep history and nature as an organism). Both disciplines see sexual orientation, preferences, and tastes as biological and evolutionary factors. Those inspired by Foucault's work, by contrast, question the existence of a natural or true human nature. Like Foucault, they prefer to speak about how particular types of knowledge about sex occur, and how these in turn inform our desires and ways of practicing and thinking about sex.

In relation to the above, we can claim that Foucault radically challenges liberal schools of thought and, in this case, liberal approaches to sexuality. Without denying the need for political action and resistance to oppression, Foucault's work has helped confront the use of essentialism* (the view that there is such a thing as an essential human nature) to demand human rights.[9] These challenges are very much in the spirit of Foucault, who preferred to contest ideas usually taken for granted by putting them into a historical context and raising questions about them.

NOTES

1   See Ann Laura Stoler, *Race and the Education of Desire: Foucault's History of Sexuality and the Colonial Order of Things* (Durham, North Carolina: Duke University Press, 1995), 1–2.

2   See Thomas Roach, "Sense and Sexuality: Foucault, Wojnarowicz, and Biopower," *Nebula: A Journal of Multidisciplinary Scholarship* 6, no. 3 (2009).

3   "Michel Foucault: Beyond Good and Evil," BFI, 1993, accessed March 6, 2016, http://www.bfi.org.uk/films-tv-people/4ce2b7c9bb0c5.

4   Thomas Hirschhorn, "24h Foucualt", October 1, 2004, accessed March 6, 2016, http://1995-2015.undo.net/it/mostra/21388.

5   See Robin Bunton and Alan Petersen, eds., *Foucault, Health and Medicine* (London: Routledge, 2002); Jennifer Radden, *The Philosophy of Psychiatry: A Companion* (Oxford: Oxford University Press, 2004), 248–9; Ann Branaman, "Contemporary Social Theory and the Sociological Study of Mental Health," in *Mental Health, Social Mirror*, eds. William R. Avison et al. (New York: Springer, 2007), 95–126; Ann Rogers and David Pilgrim, *A Sociology of Mental Health and Illness* (Maidenhead: Open University Press, 2014), 37–52.

6   Martha Nussbaum, "The Professor of Parody," *The New Republic* 22, no. 2 (1999): 38.

7   Nussbaum, "The Professor of Parody," 40.

8   Nussbaum, "The Professor of Parody," 38.

9   See Irene Diamond and Lee Quinby, eds., *Feminism & Foucault: Reflections on Resistance* (Boston: Northeastern University Press, 1988), 7.

MODULE 12
WHERE NEXT?

KEY POINTS

- Foucault's *Sexuality Vol. 1* continues to influence contemporary scholarship, most recently in debates about governance and globalization (the tightening of economic, cultural, and governmental connections across continental boundaries).

- Foucault's ideas are likely to continue being used in the discussion of gay marriage and gay rights, as well as in academic studies of social power structures across the ages.

- *Sexuality Vol. 1* marked an important moment in the history of the humanities* and social sciences,* highlighting the extent to which knowledge itself is produced, and academic analyses shaped by the cultural and historical context in which they are written.

Potential

Michel Foucault's *The History of Sexuality Vol. 1: The Will to Knowledge* has proved relevant to new social and historical situations, and to issues he could not have foreseen. For instance, the social theorists Antonio Negri* and Michael Hardt's* *Empire* (2000) uses Foucault's concepts of biopolitics* and biopower* to trace the shift from the traditional rule of kings and queens and the traditional nation-state to a world order made up of multinational corporations and transnational government organizations (such as the United Nations).*[1]

In *Sexuality Vol. 1,* Foucault argued that forces that he labeled "biopolitical" aim to regulate social life and that the language used around sexuality* was one of the most important of these forces.

> " When I read—and I know that it has been attributed
> to me—the thesis that 'knowledge is power' or 'power is
> knowledge,' I begin to laugh, since studying their *relation*
> is precisely my problem. If they were identical, I would
> not have to study them and I would be spared a lot of
> fatigue as a result. The very fact that I pose the question
> of their relation proves clearly that I do not identify
> them as the same. "
>
> Michel Foucault, as cited in Gérard Raulet. "Structuralism and
> Poststructuralism: An Interview with Michel Foucault"

Negri and Hardt modify Foucault's ideas: they argue that sexuality is less important a subject for regulating social life today, and insist instead that biopolitical control is linked to the economic processes of globalization. This change to Foucault's arguments partly reflects the fact that sexual minorities in the West are treated better than they were in the mid-1970s when *Sexuality Vol. 1* was written. Perhaps more importantly, it shows how Foucault's ideas are rich and flexible enough to examine issues (such as globalization) that were only just emerging when he was alive.

Future Directions

Foucault's text remains a vital reference in academic and popular debates on topics such as gender,* sexuality,* feminism* and gay activism. Especially in fields such as queer* theory and gender* and sexuality studies, the book enjoys high visibility and figures as a constant reference on college syllabuses and in new publications. As the cultural theorist Tamsin Spargo* notes in her book *Foucault and Queer Theory* (1999), both Foucault himself and his writing on sexuality have served as "a powerful model for many gay, lesbian and other intellectuals."[2] As such, we can safely conclude that *Sexuality*

Vol. 1 will continue to exert an influence as a key text for debates on the way sexual orientations and gender identities are defined and put into categories—and whether these categories are even necessary.

Efforts in the last decade to use Foucault's ideas in discussions over the legalization of gay marriage in the United States, for instance, suggest the lasting relevance of his ideas now and in future discussions of gay, lesbian, and transsexual* rights (the rights of those who feels that the gender they were assigned at birth is incorrect). In his "The Foucauldian-Marxist Conflict: Exploitation and Power in Gay Marriage" (2006), commentator Nick Stone notes that Foucault "would have been far more concerned [by] the pervasiveness of the current debate over gay marriage than with the issue itself, as the very nature of this debate serves as partial confirmation of his theories [regarding] repression and sexuality."[3] He suggests that *Sexuality Vol. 1* offers a way into thinking about the evolution of the debate over gay marriage, including how its supporters and opponents have framed their arguments, as well as how big the issue has become in public debate, noting, "That the national attention would be captured by the issue of homosexuality* in the midst of two foreign wars and serious economic troubles is a major validation of Foucault's thesis: that Western society cannot avoid being drawn to discuss its sexuality." [4]

The use of Foucault's concept of biopolitics also continues. Perhaps the most notable of these is the Italian philosopher Giorgio Agamben's* "Homo Sacer project," which he began writing in the mid-1990s. So far, Agamben has completed seven books in the series, including *Homo Sacer* (1995), *State of Exception* (2003), and, most recently, *The Highest Poverty: Monastic Rules and Form-of-Life* (2013). The last of these is a genealogical* study, in the spirit of Foucault, of the creation of written rules in the fourth century, and their eventual development into law. As with the discussion of Foucault's ideas in relation to gay marriage, Agamben's work shows how Foucault's ideas are readily adaptable to new issues.

Summary

Sexuality Vol. 1 is a key text in the humanities and social sciences. Foucault overturned the long-held view of eighteenth- and nineteenth-century society as sexually repressive. But he also showed how this view was merely a variation of a dominant position, promoted by scientific institutions such as psychiatry* and biology,* that had been pushing people to put sex into words since the eighteenth century. That is, he showed how the discussion around sexual liberation was a product of the very same institutions that first sought to study sexual behavior and regulate it.

Foucault's text laid the foundations for many fields of inquiry, including gender and sexuality studies, queer theory, and governmentality studies.* It deserves special attention for the central position it now occupies in various debates concerning politics, education, sexuality, and activism. It can also be seen as belonging to and influencing different fields of study, from literature and philosophy to sociology* and anthropology.*

As its title reminds us, however, *Sexuality Vol. 1* must be considered in the light of the discipline of history. Even though, as the history professor Allan Megill argues, "a gulf separates him from [the academic discipline of] history,"[5] Foucault's work stirred important and sharp debates among historians.[6] His work challenged the idea that the past can be understood in its entirety, let alone recounted in a unified way. Instead, he showed how our deeper beliefs inform our understanding of the past, leading us to interpret it in one way and not another. By revealing how sexuality has been studied by Western scientists, and by showing the categories, norms, and rules that have been established on the basis of those studies, Foucault also demonstrated the extent to which knowledge informs culture, shapes identities, and upholds power structures. These ideas, which were truly novel for their time, continue to influence academics' debates about power, governance, and knowledge.

NOTES

1   Michael Hardt and Antonio Negri, *Empire* (Harvard University Press, 2000).

2   Tamsin Spargo, *Foucault and Queer Theory* (Cambridge: Icon books, 1999), 8.

3   Nick Stone, "The Foucauldian-Marxist Conflict: Exploitation and Power in Gay Marriage," *Discoveries* 7 (2006): 66, accessed November 15, 2015, http://www.arts.cornell.edu/knight_institute/publicationsprizes/discoveries/ discoveriesspring2006/06stone.pdf.

4   Stone, "The Foucauldian-Marxist Conflict," 70.

5   Allan Megill, "The Reception of Foucault by Historians," *Journal of the History of Ideas* 48 (1987): 117.

6   Mark Poster, *Foucault, Marxism, and History: Mode of Production Versus Mode of Information* (Cambridge: Polity Press, 1984).

GLOSSARY

GLOSSARY OF TERMS

AIDS (Acquired Immune Deficiency Syndrome): an illness caused by HIV (human immunodeficiency virus) first observed in Congo in 1959 and in the United States in 1981. Foucault died of AIDS. He and his writings on sexuality influenced activists in the 1980s who sought to spread awareness of the disease and overturn the view that only gay men were at risk of catching it.

Anarchist political theory: a branch of political theory that advocates self-governance through nonhierarchical institutions sometimes referred to as stateless societies.

Androcentric: focusing on the experience of men.

Annales School: a method and style of history writing developed in France in the twentieth century mainly around the journal *Annales: Economies, Sociétés, Civilisations. Annales used social-scientific methods to focus on social rather than diplomatic or political issues.*

Anthropology: the study of humans and human behavior and their cultures. The field draws on a number of other fields in the physical, biological, and social sciences and humanities.

Anti-essentialism: the intellectual tradition that rejects the existence of a natural essence, or identity, in people or things (Foucault's claim, for example, that sexual identity is not instinctive, but socially constructed).

The Archaeology of Knowledge (1969): a book by Michel Foucault. Archaeology is the analysis of artifacts and ruins to understand past human activity and the societies from which they came. Foucault used the term in this book, and in the first half of his career, to refer to his approach to historical research: examining traces of past discourses and systems provides a way to understand the processes that have brought us to where we are today.

Ars erotica (art of pleasure): a Latin term Foucault uses to refer to the view of sex as an art form, which he distinguishes from the Western's scientific approach to sex as an object of knowledge: *scientia sexualis*.

Biological anthropology: a branch of anthropology that examines human evolution and ecology in relation to evolutionary history and biology, and that assumes human behavior is partly rooted in certain innate, hereditary, characteristics. These ideas are at odds with Foucault's theories, which assume that all human behavior is socially constructed.

Biology: a natural science that studies living things, including the function, structure, growth, evolution, taxonomy, and distribution of living organisms.

Biopolitics: Foucault's term for political strategies that aim to regulate and control the life of populations. He sees biopolitics as a typical type of governance in modern societies.

Biopower: a term Foucault coined, in *The History of Sexuality,* to describe "an explosion of numerous and diverse techniques for achieving the subjugation of bodies and the control of populations." The term describes how the state regulates its subjects by regulating, among other things, health, sexuality, heredity, and so on.

The Birth of the Clinic (1963): one of Foucault's early writings.

The book examines the history of modern medicine through the creation of the clinic in order to consider how pathologies (diseases) are categorized and how culture and customs influence our understanding of health. As with all of Foucault's work, the book is interested in how knowledge and truth are constructed.

Bourgeoisie: a term used in classical Marxist theory to refer to people in a capitalist economy who own the means of production—landowners, factory owners, and other employers who in turn wield power over workers of the lower classes (known as proletariats). The bourgeoisie are generally assumed to abuse their power and exploit the proletariat (the working people).

Capitalism: an economic system in which the means of production, trade, and industry are privately owned and conducted for private profit.

Colonialism: refers to the rule of one country by another, involving unequal power relations between the ruler (colonial power) and ruled (colony), and the exploitation of the colonies' resources to strengthen the economy of the colonizers' home country.

Cultural studies: an intellectual school that first emerged in Britain during the 1960s and then spread internationally. Cultural studies propose an anthropological reading of social relations, examining culture as a form of lived experience.

Demography: the study, usually using statistics, of the life-conditions of communities of people, be they the population of a city, a country, a neighborhood, or a specific institution such as a prison or university.

Discipline and Punish (1975): a text in which Foucault explores the transformations of the penal system in Western modernity.

Epistemology: term used to refer to the study of knowledge; the methods used to attain knowledge; and the basis of knowledge.

Essentialism: the view that all entities—animal, human being, group of people, physical object, idea—have certain qualities that are necessary to their identity and function. Foucault's work is anti-essentialist in that it questions whether there is such a thing as "human nature," or whether all humans share a specific human essence.

Eurocentrism: the tendency to believe that European culture is superior or more important than others. In scholarship, a Eurocentric work would be one that assumes a European perspective without acknowledging others.

Feminism: a series of ideologies and movements concerned with equal social, political, cultural, and economic rights for women, including equal rights in the home, workplace, education, and government.

Feminist, queer, gay, and lesbian studies: all these fields explore the ways that gender, sex, and sexual orientation are shaped by society and social norms.

Freudo-Marxism: theoretical approaches that combine Marxist critiques of capitalism with Freudian psychoanalysis. Some of the most notable Freudo-Marxist thinkers are Herbert Marcuse and Wilhelm Reich.

Gender identity: a person's individual experience of their gender—that is, of being a man or a woman, and of belonging to the category of male or female. A person might also have an ambiguous gender identity, or be uncertain of their gender identity.

Gender studies: the inquiry into the ways that gender—the sum of attributes considered to represent identities such as "male" or "female"—is constituted by society.

Genealogy: Foucault uses the German philosopher Nietzsche's idea of "genealogy" to describe his historical method. Genealogy examines concepts and practices within social settings without searching for their origin or inner truth. Instead, it examines these practices in relation to each other, and understands them to be dependent on each other—that is, influencing and shaping the outcomes of others.

Governmentality: practices of governing that aim to shape citizens' conduct instead of openly suppressing them. The term, coined by Foucault, helps us to understand how power works in modern societies.

Governmentality studies: a field that applies Foucault's concept of governmentality to understand how governance works in modern liberal societies, including in health care, in relation to migration and asylum issues, and in the arena of crime control.

Great Refusal: one of Herbert Marcuse's key concepts, it refers to opposition to and protest against unnecessary repression, and the struggle for the ultimate form of freedom—"to live without anxiety."

Hermaphrodism: a term used to refer to the presence of both, or a combination of, male and female organs in the same individual.

Heteronormativity/heterosexuality: the view that all human beings fit into distinct gender categories (man and woman) with corresponding natural roles, and that heterosexuality is the only normal, or natural, sexual orientation.

Heterosexuality: the sexual and/or romantic attraction to those of the opposite sex.

HIV: human immunodeficiency virus, the viral agent that causes the disease AIDS.

The History of Sexuality Vol. 2 (1984): the second volume of Foucault's study of sexuality, which examines the topic in ancient Greece, focusing specifically on the concept of pleasure, its social role, and its regulation.

The History of Sexuality Vol. 3 (1984): the third and last volume of Foucault's study of sexuality, which examines the topic in ancient Rome, focusing specifically on the concept of self-care.

Homosexuality: the sexual and/or romantic attraction to those of one's same sex.

Humanities: a broad term used to define academic disciplines relating to the study of human culture, including history, literature and literary criticism, anthropology, classics, geography, languages, law, music, theater, dance, philosophy, religion, and visual culture (film, drawing, sculpture, painting, gaming).

Hysteria: a term used in the nineteenth century to describe the physical display of psychological stress, most often in women. Foucault examines the origins of the term and its role in regulating, among other things, women's sexual desire.

Law of the Father: a phrase coined by the French psychoanalyst and philosopher Jacques Lacan to describe the law prohibiting incest, which ushers the child into the system of rules and prohibitions that regulate social bonds.

Leftist: a term used to refer to individuals or communities that hold left-wing political views, or to describe those views. Left-wing or leftist views tend to advocate change and reform in the interest of promoting equality.

Liberal feminism: an individualistic branch of feminism that assumes women can attain equality through personal actions and choices.

Liberalism: a term with different connotations in fields such as economics, society, and international relations. In a social sense, "liberalism" refers to the advocacy of civil liberties and individual rights, and political reform aimed at improving democracy and individual freedom; in an economic sense, it refers to the capitalist principle of market freedom.

Linguist: a student of linguistics (the study of the nature, functioning, and structure of languages).

Madness and Civilization (1964): an early work by Michel Foucault that examines the origins of the modern notion of insanity, relating it to the development of scientific thought following the Enlightenment. Foucault's ultimate point is to show the sociocultural roots of our understanding of mental illness.

Marxism: the intellectual and political movements built around the writings of the nineteenth-century philosopher and economist Karl Marx.

May 1968: a period of massive civil unrest in France that involved protests, strikes, occupations of schools and factories, and riots inspired by Marxist ideas of a more just society.

Medical gaze: a term Foucault uses to denote the dehumanizing, clinical approach that medical doctors have when treating patients, which consists of treating the body and mind as separate entities.

Middle Ages: a term used to refer to the period in European history between the fall of the Roman Empire (circa 500 C.E.) and the beginning of the Renaissance (fourteenth century).

Modernity: the intellectual response to the sociocultural changes that occurred from the late seventeenth century onwards, including industrialization, the growth of cities, the rise of the nation state, and political democracy. The concept came to be associated with the replacement of traditional values and beliefs by new ideals based on science, reason, and liberalism.

Neoliberalism: a political economic theory and practice that favors entrepreneurial freedoms, privatization, and market deregulation, while giving less attention to social welfare.

Neurology: the study of the brain and nervous system.

On the Genealogy of Morals: A Polemic (1887): a book by Friedrich Nietzsche, in which he traces the origins of moral concepts. Much of Foucault's work is based on, or elaborates, the ideas advanced in Nietzsche's text.

The Order of Things: An Archaeology of the Human Sciences (1966): a book by Michel Foucault that (borrowing the language of archaeology) seeks to excavate the origins of the human sciences and, in particular, sociology and psychology. As with Foucault's other works, it is above all concerned with how knowledge is constructed and our assumptions about truth; however, it differs from his late work in its specifically structuralist approach.

Orthodox Marxism: refers to narrow interpretations of Marx, mostly related to the prominent role that economics plays in social relations.

Pathology: a broad term for any psychological or physical medical disorder or suffering. Pathological behavior refers to behavior that reflects an underlying mental disorder. Much of Foucault's work was concerned with how pathologies are defined and what those definitions say about the surrounding culture.

Patriarchy: social organizations (governments, families, and other communities) ruled by males, in which descent is reckoned through the male line, and children are given the father's last name.

Pedagogy: the practice of teaching and the theories or principles on which education is based.

Phenomenology: a branch of philosophy that developed in the eighteenth century. It studies the structures that inform our experience and our consciousness of the world around us, and the role that perception plays in the way we relate to the world.

Polymorphous: something that assumes, has, or occurs in different or varying forms, characters, or styles. Foucault claims that power is polymorphous in that it assumes different forms.

Positivism: a philosophical school that holds that what one observes can be a legitimate source of human knowledge. By putting emphasis on the empirical (that which is based on experiment or observation), and on what is experienced as holding a particular "truth," positivist scholarship generally avoids looking at how subjectivities are mediated and defined by culture, ideology, and language.

Postcolonial studies: an academic discipline that studies the effects of colonialism and imperialism on once-colonized cultures and populations, before or after political "independence." It draws from a range of disciplines and schools of thought, especially from poststructuralism, critical theory, Marxist theory, and anthropology.

Post-Marxism: a social theory and philosophy grounded in Marxism that extends, reverses, or modifies it. Contemporary post-Marxists who often employ Foucault's arguments include Ernesto Laclau, Chantal Mouffe, and Antonio Negri.

Poststructuralism: a label invented to refer to the work of a mainly French group of theorists and philosophers of the 1960s and 1970s who regarded social structures and categories as basically unstable. Although Foucault was often thought of as a poststructuralist, he rejected the label.

Prison Information Group: a group founded in 1971 in France that attempted to bring radio and newspapers into prisons to expose the conditions. It published four journals attempting to "turn the prison inside out," publishing information that attempted to make prison officials rather than prisoners the targets of unwanted attention.

Psychiatry: the branch of medicine that deals in the study, treatment, and prevention of mental disorders.

Psychoanalysis: a theory and method conceived by Sigmund Freud in the late nineteenth century that seeks to understand the human psyche and treat mental disorders.

Psychology: an academic and applied discipline dealing with the study and treatment of mental behavior and mental functions.

Queer theory: an academic field that emerged in North American humanities departments in the 1990s and then spread mainly throughout the English-speaking academic world. Queer theory wishes to disturb traditional sexual and other categories.

Repressive hypothesis: the title of one of the chapters in Michel Foucault's *The History of Sexuality Vol. 1,* and a term he uses throughout the book to describe a particular set of beliefs regarding sexuality's role throughout history, which were advanced by Freudo-Marxist academics in the 1960s and 1970s, as well as by post-May 1968 advocates of sexual liberation.

Roman Catholic confession: a religious rite in which an individual tells a priest his or her sins—things they have done that go against Christian teachings—and ask for God's forgiveness.

Roman Catholicism: a broad term used to define traditions specific to the Roman Catholic Church, including (but not limited to) their doctrine, ethics, and theology.

Repressive hypothesis: the title of one of the chapters in Michel Foucault's *The History of Sexuality Vol. 1,* and a term he uses to define the scientific study of sex and sexuality in the modern era (late seventeenth century to the present), that led to putting sexual acts and feelings into various categories and the regulation of sexuality and sexual behavior.

Sexuality studies: an academic field that explores the ways that sexual identities are constituted in society at large, in spheres such as cinema, art, popular culture, literature, and politics.

Sexual orientation: a term used to refer to a person's sexual identity in relation to the gender to which they are attracted. Heterosexual, homosexual, and bisexual are all sexual orientations.

Social sciences: a broad term that groups academic disciplines examining society and human relationships within society, including economics, history, law, psychology, sociology, political science, education, geography, and anthropology.

Sociology: the academic study of social behavior. The discipline examines the origins and development of social relations, their different modes of organization, and different social institutions.

Structuralism: a theoretical approach arguing that elements of culture become intelligible if studied in relation to the larger structures and systems to which they belong. It originated in the linguistics of Ferdinand de Saussure and was later developed by, among others, the anthropologist Claude Lévi-Strauss.

Subjectivity: a concept used to explain differences between individuals (including tastes, opinions, values, and beliefs), and to account for the distance between a person's views and those of their surrounding community. In philosophy, the concept is crucial to the discussion of why people are so different in the way they interpret and relate to the world around them.

Theology: the systematic study of religious ideas, usually conducted through readings of scripture.

Transsexual: a person who feels that the gender they were assigned at birth (on the basis of their genitals) is incorrect. A transsexual may choose to undergo gender-reassignment surgery and hormone therapy to become the gender they feel they are.

United Nations: an international body instituted following World War II designed to foster communication, cooperation, and security between nations; its headquarters is in New York.

Victorian morality: the moral values that prevailed at the time of Queen Victoria's reign in Great Britain from 1837 to 1901. These moral values involved strict rules of social conduct, like sexual constraints and a prohibition against scandalous language.

Vietnam War (1955–1975): a conflict fought in Vietnam that also involved Laos and Cambodia. It pitted the nationalist South Vietnam against the communist North Vietnam. Opposition to France's role in the war was among the causes of unrest in the events leading up to May 1968.

Will to power: an important concept developed by Friedrich Nietzsche that he used to describe what he thought was the motivating force in humans: ambition and the desire to achieve the highest possible position available to them.

World War I (1914–1918): A global war between two alliances: the Central Powers (Germany and Austria-Hungary) and the Allies (the Russian Empire, the British Empire, and France).

PEOPLE MENTIONED IN THE TEXT

Giorgio Agamben (b. 1942) is an important contemporary Italian philosopher and political theorist working in the fields of linguistics, law, and politics. Some of his most well-known works are *Homo Sacer* (1998) and *State of Exception* (2005).

Louis Althusser (1918–90) was a French Marxist philosopher who is often associated today with the school of structuralism. However, Althusser was critical of certain aspects of structuralist thought, and spent his life supporting the central tenets of Marxism. Foucault was greatly influenced by Althusser's work.

Judith Butler (b. 1956) is an influential American theorist and academic whose work has significantly shaped fields such as feminist and queer theory. Her most notable books include *Gender Trouble* (1990) and *Bodies That Matter* (1993).

James Clifford (b. 1945) is an American anthropologist.

Jacques Derrida (1930–2004) was a French philosopher best known for his work in the development of "deconstruction," a form of semiotic analysis, and for his involvement in the schools of structuralism and poststructuralism. Derrida and Foucault hugely disagreed in their critical approaches, and it has been said that Foucault wrote some of his books as a direct response to Derrida's criticisms.

Epictetus (55–135 C.E.) was a Greek-speaking philosopher who lived in Rome, and who championed philosophy as a way of life, not just a theoretical discipline. Foucault makes frequent reference to Epictetus's ideas about morality, death, independence, and selfhood in *The History of Sexuality Vol. 3*.

Sigmund Freud (1856–1939) was an Austrian neurologist who pioneered the view that human actions are driven in large part by unconscious desires and primordial urges. He is the founder of psychoanalysis.

David M. Halperin (b. 1952) is an American scholar specializing in the fields of queer theory, queer studies, critical theory, visual culture, and material culture. He is best known for his book *One Hundred Years of Homosexuality* (1990), in which he argues the historical significance of the use of the term "homosexual" by Richard von Krafft-Ebing in the study of sexual pathologies, *Psycopathia Sexualis*, which was translated into English in 1892. Halperin has also written extensively on Foucault and his influence on queer studies.

Michael Hardt (b. 1960) is an American Marxist/post-Marxist literary theorist and political philosopher best known for coauthoring *Empire* (2000) with Antonio Negri, a book that applies Foucault's concepts of biopower and biopolitics to examine how power operates in the post-Cold War, globalized economy.

Thomas Hirschhorn (b. 1957) is a Swiss artist known for his politically charged art installations that often pay tribute to seminal left-wing thinkers. To date he has created works inspired by Antonio Gramsci, Gilles Deleuze, and Michel Foucault. His *24h Foucault,* an art installation featuring (among other things) a library, shop, bar, and auditorium, sought to create a space for viewers akin to the inside of Foucault's brain.

Jean Hyppolite (1907–68) was a French philosopher and follower of Georg Hegel and the German philosophical movement, and a prominent figure in French thinking in the mid-twentieth century. Foucault studied under him and was profoundly shaped by his ideas on the relationship between history and philosophy.

Jacques Lacan (1901–81) was a French psychoanalyst and psychiatrist best known for advocating a "return to Freud" through a close reading of his texts and a redress of the way in which Freud's theories had been misunderstood and perverted by his followers, especially in the United States. Lacanian psychoanalysis had a profound influence on French philosophy and feminist theory.

Ernesto Laclau (1935–2014) was an Argentine post-Marxist political theorist. He is best known for *Hegemony and Socialist Strategy* (1985), which he coauthored with Chantal Mouffe, and for his first book, *Politics and Ideology in Marxist Theory* (1977). Laclau was greatly influenced by Foucault's writings on power.

Claude Lévi-Strauss (1908–2009) was a French ethnologist and anthropologist, and is frequently cited as the "father of modern anthropology." His work is based on the application of the structural linguistic theories of Ferdinand de Saussure to anthropology.

Herbert Marcuse (1898–1979) was an influential American-based German philosopher and prominent member of the Frankfurt School working at the intersection of Marxism and psychoanalysis. His best known works include *Eros and Civilization* (1955) and *One-Dimensional Man* (1964).

Biddy Martin (b. 1951) is an American writer and intellectual known for her writings on feminism and queer theory—most notably, *Femininity Played Straight: The Significance of Being Lesbian* (1996). Martin has been critical of Foucault's work, arguing that his views on sexuality are androcentric, and do not lend themselves to feminist applications.

Karl Marx (1818–83) was a German political philosopher and economist whose analysis of class relations under capitalism and articulation of a more egalitarian system provided the basis for communism. Together with Friedrich Engels (1820–1895), Marx wrote *The Communist Manifesto* (1848). He articulated his full theory of production and class relations in *Das Kapital* (1867).

Maurice Merleau-Ponty (1908–61) was a French phenomenological philosopher and writer, and the only major philosopher of his time to incorporate descriptive psychology in his work. This influenced later phenomenologists, who went on to use cognitive science and psychology in their studies.

Chantal Mouffe (b. 1943) is a Belgian political theorist best known for developing, together with Ernesto Laclau, the school of discourse analysis—an approach to post-Marxist political inquiry that draws on poststructuralist ideas, including Foucault's. She and Laclau coauthored *Hegemony and Socialist Strategy* (1977), the text credited with laying the grounds of discourse analysis.

Antonio Negri (b. 1933) is an Italian Marxist/post-Marxist philosopher best known for coauthoring *Empire* (2000) with Michael Hardt. Negri uses Foucault's concepts of biopower and biopolitics in much of his writing.

Friedrich Nietzsche (1844–1900) was a prominent German philosopher who radically questioned concepts such as religion, morality, and truth.

Martha Nussbaum (b. 1947) is an American philosopher. She is professor of law and ethics at the University of Chicago.

Monique Plaza is a French feminist writer and thinker, and cofounder of the influential French journal *Questiones Feministes*, which first published in 1980. Plaza was an outspoken critic of Foucault.

Plutarch (46–120 C.E.) was a Greek essayist, historian, and biographer. Foucault wrote about Plutarch's work on love and sex in *The History of Sexuality Vol. 3*.

Wilhelm Reich (1897–1957) was a radical Austrian psychoanalyst who wrote extensively on the effects of sexual repression. His most notable works include *The Mass Psychology of Fascism* (1933) and *The Sexual Revolution* (1936).

Nikolas Rose (b. 1947) is an influential British social theorist and sociologist who has written on mental health policy and risk, the sociology and history of psychiatry, and the social implications of new psychopharmacological developments in the area of mental health. He is best known for his writings on Foucault and for reviving interest in Foucault's concept of governmentality in the Anglophone world.

Ferdinand de Saussure (1857–1913) was a Swiss linguist whose ideas on structure in language laid the foundation for the linguistic sciences in the twentieth century.

Alan D. Schrift is an American professor of nineteenth- and twentieth-century French and German philosophy at Grinnell College, Iowa. He has written extensively on Foucault.

Eve Sedgwick (1950–2009) was an influential American theorist and university professor in the fields of queer theory and gender studies. Her most celebrated work is *Epistemology of the Closet* (1990).

Seneca (4 B.C.E.–65 C.E.) was Roman philosopher, tutor to the emperor Nero, and proponent of the philosophical school of Stoicism; Foucault discussed him in *The History of Sexuality Vol. 3*. Foucault's work on Seneca's idea of the "care of the self" caused scholars to revise their assessment of the work.

Tamsin Spargo is a cultural historian specializing in queer theory, queer culture, gender, and countercultural literature.

Gayatri Chakravorty Spivak (b. 1942) is an Indian theorist and philosopher, whose work has proved extremely influential within the discipline of postcolonial studies. One of her most widely read texts is the essay "Can the Subaltern Speak?" (1988).

Ann Stoler (b. 1949) is an American anthropologist best known for her writings on the sexual politics of empire (how sexuality and gender are treated under colonial rule), as well as issues of colonial governance. She was among the first academics to point out Foucault's failure to mention colonialism as a decisive factor in his account of sexuality in modern Western culture.

Fathi Triki (b. 1947) is a French philosopher and emeritus professor at the University of Tunisia. He studied under Foucault and was greatly influenced by his ideas.

Carl Westphal (1833–90) was a German psychiatrist best known for coining the term "agoraphobia"—the fear of large, open spaces—and credited, by Foucault, for creating the term "homosexual," which influenced the modern definition of homosexuality as something tied to one's identity. Westphal considered homosexuality to be a psychiatric disorder.

David Wojnarowicz (1954–92) was a gay artist, writer, filmmaker, photographer, and AIDS activist best known for his involvement in the New York City art scene of the 1970s and 1980s, and for his often controversial art installations that sought to challenge the stigmatization of homosexuality and AIDS. He is frequently discussed by queer theorists in relation to Foucault's work.

WORKS CITED

WORKS CITED

Afary, Janet, and Kevin B. Anderson. "Foucault, Gender and Male Homosexualities in Mediterranean and Muslim Society." In *Foucault and the Iranian Revolution: Gender and the Seductions of Islamism,* 138–62. Chicago: Chicago University Press, 2005.

Agamben, Giorgio. *The Highest Poverty: Monastic Rules and Form-of-Life.* Translated by Adam Kotsko. Stanford: Stanford University Press, 2013.

——— *Homo Sacer: Sovereign Power and Bare Life.* Translated by Daniel Heller-Roazen. Stanford: Stanford University Press, 1998.

——— *State of Exception.* Translated by Kevin Attell. Chicago: University of Chicago Press, 2005.

Allen, Amy. "Foucault, Feminism and the Self: The Politics of Personal Transformation." In *Feminism and the Final Foucault*, edited by Dianna Taylor and Karen Vintges, 235–57. Chicago: University of Illinois Press, 2004.

Ball, Kelly H. "'More or Less Raped': Foucault, Causality, and Feminist Critiques of Sexual Violence." *philoSOPHIA* 3, no.1 (2013): 52–68.

Branaman, Ann. "Contemporary Social Theory and the Sociological Study of Mental Health." In *Mental Health, Social Mirror,* edited by William R. Avison, Jane D. McLeod and Bernice A. Pescosolido, 95–126. New York: Springer, 2007.

Bunton, Robin, and Alan Petersen, eds. *Foucault, Health and Medicine.* London: Routledge, 2002.

Butler, Judith. *Bodies That Matter*. London: Routledge, 1993.

——— *Gender Trouble.* London: Routledge, 1990.

Carrette, Jeremy R. *Foucault and Religion: Spiritual Corporality and Political Spirituality.* London: Routledge, 2000.

Cavallaro, Dani. *French Feminist Theory: An Introduction.* London: Continuum, 2003.

Clark, Elizabeth A. "Foucault, The Fathers and Sex." *Journal of the American Academy of Religion* 56, no .4 (1988): 619–41.

Clifford, James. *The Predicament of Culture: Twentieth-Century Ethnography, Literature, and Art.* Cambridge, Mass: Harvard University Press, 1988.

Defert, Daniel. "Chronology." In *A Companion to Foucault*, edited by Christopher Falzon, Timothy O'Leary and Jana Sawicki. Chichester: Wiley & Sons, 2013.

Diamond, Irene, and Lee Quinby. *Feminism & Foucault: Reflections on Resistance.* Boston: Northeastern University Press, 1988.

Dosse, Francois. *History of Structuralism. Volume II. The Sign Sets 1967– Present.* Translated by Deborah Glassman. Minneapolis: University of Minnesota Press, 1998.

Dreyfus, Hubert, and Paul Rabinow, eds. *Michel Foucault: Beyond Structuralism and Hermeneutics.* Chicago: University of Chicago Press, 1983.

Foucault, Michel. *The Archaeology of Knowledge (and the Discourse on Language).* Translated by A. M. Sheridan-Smith. London: Tavistock Publications Limited, 1972.

——— *The Birth of the Clinic: An Archaeology of Medical Perception.* Translated by A. M. Sheridan-Smith. London: Routledge, 2003.

——— *Discipline and Punish: The Birth of the Prison.* Translated by Alan Sheridan-Smith. New York: Random House, 1977.

——— "The Ethics of the Concern for Self as a Practice of Freedom." Translated by P. Aranaov and D. McGrawth. In *Michel Foucault: Ethics, Subjectivity and Truth*, edited by Paul Rabinow, 281–302. New York: The New Press, 1997.

——— *"La Folie Encirclé."* *Change Collective* (Paris: 1977).

——— *The History of Sexuality Vol. 1: The Will to Knowledge.* Translated by Robert Hurley. London: Penguin Books, 1998.

——— *The History of Sexuality Vol. 2: The Use of Pleasure.* Translated by Robert Hurley. New York: Random House Digital, Inc., 2012.

——— *The History of Sexuality Vol. 3: The Care of the Self.* Translated by Robert Hurley. New York: Random House Digital, Inc., 2012.

——— *Madness and Civilization: A History of Insanity in the Age of Reason.* Translated by Richard Howard. London: Vintage, 2006.

——— *The Order of Things: An Archaeology of the Human Sciences.* London: Routledge, 2001).

——— *Power/knowledge: Selected Interviews and Other Writings: 1972– 1977.* Edited by Colin Gordon. Translated by Colin Gordon, Leo Marshall, John Mepham and Kate Soper. New York: Random House, 1980.

——— "Sexual Choice, Sexual Act." Translated by James O'Higgins. In *Michel Foucault: Ethics, Subjectivity and Truth*, edited by Paul Rabinow. New York: The New Press, 1997.

Fraser, Nancy. "From Discipline to Flexibilization? Rereading Foucault in the

Shadow of Globalization," *Constellations* 10, no. 2 (2003): 160–71.

Halperin, David. *One Hundred Years of Homosexuality: and other Essays on Greek Love.* London: Routledge, 1990.

——— *Saint Foucault: Towards a Gay Hagiography.* New York: Oxford University Press, 1995.

Hardt, Michael, and Antonio Negri. *Empire.* Cambridge: Harvard University Press, 2000.

Larmour, David H. J., Paul Allen and Charles Platter. "Situating the *History of Sexuality.*" In *Rethinking Sexuality: Foucault and Classical Antiquity,* edited by David H. J. Larmour, Paul Allen Miller, and Charles Platter, 3–41. Princeton, New Jersey: Princeton University Press, 1998.

Larner, Wendy. "Neo-liberalism: Policy, Ideology, Governmentality." *Studies in Political Economy* 63 (2000): 5–25.

Leonard, Diana, and Lisa Adkins. "Reconstructing French Feminism: Commodification, Materialism and Sex." In *Sex in Question: French Materialist Feminism*, edited by Diana Leonard and Lisa Adkins, 1–23. London: Taylor & Francis, 1996.

Macey, David. *The Lives of Michel Foucault.* New York: Pantheon, 1993.

Marcuse, Herbert. *Eros and Civilization: A Philosophical Inquiry into Freud.* Boston: Beacon Press, 1974.

——— *One-Dimensional Man: Studies in the Ideology of Advanced Industrial Society.* London: Routledge, 2002.

Martin, Biddy. "Feminism, Criticism, and Foucault." *New German Critique* 27 (1982): 3–30.

McWhorter, Ladelle. *Bodies and Pleasures: Foucault and the Politics of Sexual Normalization.* Bloomington: Indiana University Press, 1999.

Megill, Allan. "The Reception of Foucault by Historians." *Journal of the History of Ideas* 48 (1987): 117–41.

Nietzsche, Friedrich. *On the Genealogy of Morals and Ecce Homo.* New York: Random House, 2010 .

——— *The Will to Power.* New York: Random House, 2011.

Nussbaum, Martha. "The Professor of Parody." *The New Republic* 22, no. 2 (1999): 37–45.

Plaza, Monique. "Our Costs and Their Benefits." In *Sex in Question: French Materialist Feminism*, edited by Diana Leonard and Lisa Adkins, 183–94. London: Taylor & Francis, 1996.

Poster, Mark. *Foucault, Marxism, and History: Mode of Production Versus Mode of Information.* Cambridge: Polity Press, 1984.

Rabinow, Paul. "Series Preface." In *Michel Foucault: Ethics, Subjectivity and Truth,* edited by Paul Rabinow. New York: The New Press, 1997.

Radden, Jennifer, ed. *The Philosophy of Psychiatry: A Companion.* Oxford: Oxford University Press, 2004.

Raulet, Gérard. "Structuralism and Post-structuralism: An Interview with Michel Foucault." *Telos* 55 (1983): 195–211. Accessed 16 October 2015. doi: 10.3817/0383055195.

Reich, Wilhelm. *The Mass Psychology of Fascism.* New York: Farrar, Straus & Giroux, 1970.

Roach, Thomas. "Sense and Sexuality: Foucault, Wojnarowicz, and Biopower." *Nebula: A Journal of Multidisciplinary Scholarship* 6, no. 3 (2009): 155–73.

Rogers, Ann, and David Pilgrim. *A Sociology of Mental Health and Illness.* Maidenhead: Open University Press.

Schrift, Alan D. *Nietzsche's French Legacy: A Genealogy of Poststructuralism.* London: Routledge, 1995.

Soper, Kate. "Productive Contradictions." In *Up Against Foucault: Explorations of Some Tensions Between Foucault and Feminism,* edited by Caroline Ramazanoglu, 29–51. New York: Routledge, 1993.

Spargo, Tamsin. *Foucault and Queer Theory.* Cambridge: Icon books, 1999.

Stoler, Ann Laura. *Race and the Education of Desire: Foucault's History of Sexuality and the Colonial Order of Things.* Durham, North Carolina: Duke University Press, 1995.

Stone, Nick. "The Foucauldian-Marxist Conflict: Exploitation and Power in Gay Marriage." *Discoveries* 7 (2006): 65–72. Accessed November 15, 2015. http://www.arts.cornell.edu/knight_institute/publicationsprizes/discoveries/discoveriesspring2006/06stone.pdf.

Sullivan, Nikki. *A Critical Introduction to Queer Theory.* New York: NYU Press, 2003.

THE MACAT LIBRARY
BY DISCIPLINE

AFRICANA STUDIES

Chinua Achebe's *An Image of Africa: Racism in Conrad's Heart of Darkness*
W. E. B. Du Bois's *The Souls of Black Folk*
Zora Neale Huston's *Characteristics of Negro Expression*
Martin Luther King Jr's *Why We Can't Wait*
Toni Morrison's *Playing in the Dark: Whiteness in the American Literary Imagination*

ANTHROPOLOGY

Arjun Appadurai's *Modernity at Large: Cultural Dimensions of Globalisation*
Philippe Ariès's *Centuries of Childhood*
Franz Boas's *Race, Language and Culture*
Kim Chan & Renée Mauborgne's *Blue Ocean Strategy*
Jared Diamond's *Guns, Germs & Steel: the Fate of Human Societies*
Jared Diamond's *Collapse: How Societies Choose to Fail or Survive*
E. E. Evans-Pritchard's *Witchcraft, Oracles and Magic Among the Azande*
James Ferguson's *The Anti-Politics Machine*
Clifford Geertz's *The Interpretation of Cultures*
David Graeber's *Debt: the First 5000 Years*
Karen Ho's *Liquidated: An Ethnography of Wall Street*
Geert Hofstede's *Culture's Consequences: Comparing Values, Behaviors, Institutes and Organizations across Nations*
Claude Lévi-Strauss's *Structural Anthropology*
Jay Macleod's *Ain't No Makin' It: Aspirations and Attainment in a Low-Income Neighborhood*
Saba Mahmood's *The Politics of Piety: The Islamic Revival and the Feminist Subjec*t
Marcel Mauss's *The Gift*

BUSINESS

Jean Lave & Etienne Wenger's *Situated Learning*
Theodore Levitt's *Marketing Myopia*
Burton G. Malkiel's *A Random Walk Down Wall Street*
Douglas McGregor's *The Human Side of Enterprise*
Michael Porter's *Competitive Strategy: Creating and Sustaining Superior Performance*
John Kotter's *Leading Change*
C. K. Prahalad & Gary Hamel's *The Core Competence of the Corporation*

CRIMINOLOGY

Michelle Alexander's *The New Jim Crow: Mass Incarceration in the Age of Colorblindness*
Michael R. Gottfredson & Travis Hirschi's *A General Theory of Crime*
Richard Herrnstein & Charles A. Murray's *The Bell Curve: Intelligence and Class Structure in American Life*
Elizabeth Loftus's *Eyewitness Testimony*
Jay Macleod's *Ain't No Makin' It: Aspirations and Attainment in a Low-Income Neighborhood*
Philip Zimbardo's *The Lucifer Effect*

ECONOMICS

Janet Abu-Lughod's *Before European Hegemony*
Ha-Joon Chang's *Kicking Away the Ladder*
David Brion Davis's *The Problem of Slavery in the Age of Revolution*
Milton Friedman's *The Role of Monetary Policy*
Milton Friedman's *Capitalism and Freedom*
David Graeber's *Debt: the First 5000 Years*
Friedrich Hayek's *The Road to Serfdom*
Karen Ho's *Liquidated: An Ethnography of Wall Street*

John Maynard Keynes's *The General Theory of Employment, Interest and Money*
Charles P. Kindleberger's *Manias, Panics and Crashes*
Robert Lucas's *Why Doesn't Capital Flow from Rich to Poor Countries?*
Burton G. Malkiel's *A Random Walk Down Wall Street*
Thomas Robert Malthus's *An Essay on the Principle of Population*
Karl Marx's *Capital*
Thomas Piketty's *Capital in the Twenty-First Century*
Amartya Sen's *Development as Freedom*
Adam Smith's *The Wealth of Nations*
Nassim Nicholas Taleb's *The Black Swan: The Impact of the Highly Improbable*
Amos Tversky's & Daniel Kahneman's *Judgment under Uncertainty: Heuristics and Biases*
Mahbub Ul Haq's *Reflections on Human Development*
Max Weber's *The Protestant Ethic and the Spirit of Capitalism*

FEMINISM AND GENDER STUDIES

Judith Butler's *Gender Trouble*
Simone De Beauvoir's *The Second Sex*
Michel Foucault's *History of Sexuality*
Betty Friedan's *The Feminine Mystique*
Saba Mahmood's *The Politics of Piety: The Islamic Revival and the Feminist Subject*
Joan Wallach Scott's *Gender and the Politics of History*
Mary Wollstonecraft's *A Vindication of the Rights of Women*
Virginia Woolf's *A Room of One's Own*

GEOGRAPHY

The Brundtland Report's *Our Common Future*
Rachel Carson's *Silent Spring*
Charles Darwin's *On the Origin of Species*
James Ferguson's *The Anti-Politics Machine*
Jane Jacobs's *The Death and Life of Great American Cities*
James Lovelock's *Gaia: A New Look at Life on Earth*
Amartya Sen's *Development as Freedom*
Mathis Wackernagel & William Rees's *Our Ecological Footprint*

HISTORY

Janet Abu-Lughod's *Before European Hegemony*
Benedict Anderson's *Imagined Communities*
Bernard Bailyn's *The Ideological Origins of the American Revolution*
Hanna Batatu's *The Old Social Classes And The Revolutionary Movements Of Iraq*
Christopher Browning's *Ordinary Men: Reserve Police Batallion 101 and the Final Solution in Poland*
Edmund Burke's *Reflections on the Revolution in France*
William Cronon's *Nature's Metropolis: Chicago And The Great West*
Alfred W. Crosby's *The Columbian Exchange*
Hamid Dabashi's *Iran: A People Interrupted*
David Brion Davis's *The Problem of Slavery in the Age of Revolution*
Nathalie Zemon Davis's *The Return of Martin Guerre*
Jared Diamond's *Guns, Germs & Steel: the Fate of Human Societies*
Frank Dikotter's *Mao's Great Famine*
John W Dower's *War Without Mercy: Race And Power In The Pacific War*
W. E. B. Du Bois's *The Souls of Black Folk*
Richard J. Evans's *In Defence of History*
Lucien Febvre's *The Problem of Unbelief in the 16th Century*
Sheila Fitzpatrick's *Everyday Stalinism*

Eric Foner's *Reconstruction: America's Unfinished Revolution, 1863-1877*
Michel Foucault's *Discipline and Punish*
Michel Foucault's *History of Sexuality*
Francis Fukuyama's *The End of History and the Last Man*
John Lewis Gaddis's *We Now Know: Rethinking Cold War History*
Ernest Gellner's *Nations and Nationalism*
Eugene Genovese's *Roll, Jordan, Roll: The World the Slaves Made*
Carlo Ginzburg's *The Night Battles*
Daniel Goldhagen's *Hitler's Willing Executioners*
Jack Goldstone's *Revolution and Rebellion in the Early Modern World*
Antonio Gramsci's *The Prison Notebooks*
Alexander Hamilton, John Jay & James Madison's *The Federalist Papers*
Christopher Hill's *The World Turned Upside Down*
Carole Hillenbrand's *The Crusades: Islamic Perspectives*
Thomas Hobbes's *Leviathan*
Eric Hobsbawm's *The Age Of Revolution*
John A. Hobson's *Imperialism: A Study*
Albert Hourani's *History of the Arab Peoples*
Samuel P. Huntington's *The Clash of Civilizations and the Remaking of World Order*
C. L. R. James's *The Black Jacobins*
Tony Judt's *Postwar: A History of Europe Since 1945*
Ernst Kantorowicz's *The King's Two Bodies: A Study in Medieval Political Theology*
Paul Kennedy's *The Rise and Fall of the Great Powers*
Ian Kershaw's *The "Hitler Myth": Image and Reality in the Third Reich*
John Maynard Keynes's *The General Theory of Employment, Interest and Money*
Charles P. Kindleberger's *Manias, Panics and Crashes*
Martin Luther King Jr's *Why We Can't Wait*
Henry Kissinger's *World Order: Reflections on the Character of Nations and the Course of History*
Thomas Kuhn's *The Structure of Scientific Revolutions*
Georges Lefebvre's *The Coming of the French Revolution*
John Locke's *Two Treatises of Government*
Niccolò Machiavelli's *The Prince*
Thomas Robert Malthus's *An Essay on the Principle of Population*
Mahmood Mamdani's *Citizen and Subject: Contemporary Africa And The Legacy Of Late Colonialism*
Karl Marx's *Capital*
Stanley Milgram's *Obedience to Authority*
John Stuart Mill's *On Liberty*
Thomas Paine's *Common Sense*
Thomas Paine's *Rights of Man*
Geoffrey Parker's *Global Crisis: War, Climate Change and Catastrophe in the Seventeenth Century*
Jonathan Riley-Smith's *The First Crusade and the Idea of Crusading*
Jean-Jacques Rousseau's *The Social Contract*
Joan Wallach Scott's *Gender and the Politics of History*
Theda Skocpol's *States and Social Revolutions*
Adam Smith's *The Wealth of Nations*
Timothy Snyder's *Bloodlands: Europe Between Hitler and Stalin*
Sun Tzu's *The Art of War*
Keith Thomas's *Religion and the Decline of Magic*
Thucydides's *The History of the Peloponnesian War*
Frederick Jackson Turner's *The Significance of the Frontier in American History*
Odd Arne Westad's *The Global Cold War: Third World Interventions And The Making Of Our Times*

The Macat Library By Discipline

LITERATURE

Chinua Achebe's *An Image of Africa: Racism in Conrad's Heart of Darkness*
Roland Barthes's *Mythologies*
Homi K. Bhabha's *The Location of Culture*
Judith Butler's *Gender Trouble*
Simone De Beauvoir's *The Second Sex*
Ferdinand De Saussure's *Course in General Linguistics*
T. S. Eliot's *The Sacred Wood: Essays on Poetry and Criticism*
Zora Neale Huston's *Characteristics of Negro Expression*
Toni Morrison's *Playing in the Dark: Whiteness in the American Literary Imagination*
Edward Said's *Orientalism*
Gayatri Chakravorty Spivak's *Can the Subaltern Speak?*
Mary Wollstonecraft's *A Vindication of the Rights of Women*
Virginia Woolf's *A Room of One's Own*

PHILOSOPHY

Elizabeth Anscombe's *Modern Moral Philosophy*
Hannah Arendt's *The Human Condition*
Aristotle's *Metaphysics*
Aristotle's *Nicomachean Ethics*
Edmund Gettier's *Is Justified True Belief Knowledge?*
Georg Wilhelm Friedrich Hegel's *Phenomenology of Spirit*
David Hume's *Dialogues Concerning Natural Religion*
David Hume's *The Enquiry for Human Understanding*
Immanuel Kant's *Religion within the Boundaries of Mere Reason*
Immanuel Kant's *Critique of Pure Reason*
Søren Kierkegaard's *The Sickness Unto Death*
Søren Kierkegaard's *Fear and Trembling*
C. S. Lewis's *The Abolition of Man*
Alasdair MacIntyre's *After Virtue*
Marcus Aurelius's *Meditations*
Friedrich Nietzsche's *On the Genealogy of Morality*
Friedrich Nietzsche's *Beyond Good and Evil*
Plato's *Republic*
Plato's *Symposium*
Jean-Jacques Rousseau's *The Social Contract*
Gilbert Ryle's *The Concept of Mind*
Baruch Spinoza's *Ethics*
Sun Tzu's *The Art of War*
Ludwig Wittgenstein's *Philosophical Investigations*

POLITICS

Benedict Anderson's *Imagined Communities*
Aristotle's *Politics*
Bernard Bailyn's *The Ideological Origins of the American Revolution*
Edmund Burke's *Reflections on the Revolution in France*
John C. Calhoun's *A Disquisition on Government*
Ha-Joon Chang's *Kicking Away the Ladder*
Hamid Dabashi's *Iran: A People Interrupted*
Hamid Dabashi's *Theology of Discontent: The Ideological Foundation of the Islamic Revolution in Iran*
Robert Dahl's *Democracy and its Critics*
Robert Dahl's *Who Governs?*
David Brion Davis's *The Problem of Slavery in the Age of Revolution*

Alexis De Tocqueville's *Democracy in America*
James Ferguson's *The Anti-Politics Machine*
Frank Dikotter's *Mao's Great Famine*
Sheila Fitzpatrick's *Everyday Stalinism*
Eric Foner's *Reconstruction: America's Unfinished Revolution, 1863-1877*
Milton Friedman's *Capitalism and Freedom*
Francis Fukuyama's *The End of History and the Last Man*
John Lewis Gaddis's *We Now Know: Rethinking Cold War History*
Ernest Gellner's *Nations and Nationalism*
David Graeber's *Debt: the First 5000 Years*
Antonio Gramsci's *The Prison Notebooks*
Alexander Hamilton, John Jay & James Madison's *The Federalist Papers*
Friedrich Hayek's *The Road to Serfdom*
Christopher Hill's *The World Turned Upside Down*
Thomas Hobbes's *Leviathan*
John A. Hobson's *Imperialism: A Study*
Samuel P. Huntington's *The Clash of Civilizations and the Remaking of World Order*
Tony Judt's *Postwar: A History of Europe Since 1945*
David C. Kang's *China Rising: Peace, Power and Order in East Asia*
Paul Kennedy's *The Rise and Fall of Great Powers*
Robert Keohane's *After Hegemony*
Martin Luther King Jr.'s *Why We Can't Wait*
Henry Kissinger's *World Order: Reflections on the Character of Nations and the Course of History*
John Locke's *Two Treatises of Government*
Niccolò Machiavelli's *The Prince*
Thomas Robert Malthus's *An Essay on the Principle of Population*
Mahmood Mamdani's *Citizen and Subject: Contemporary Africa And The Legacy Of Late Colonialism*
Karl Marx's *Capital*
John Stuart Mill's *On Liberty*
John Stuart Mill's *Utilitarianism*
Hans Morgenthau's *Politics Among Nations*
Thomas Paine's *Common Sense*
Thomas Paine's *Rights of Man*
Thomas Piketty's *Capital in the Twenty-First Century*
Robert D. Putnam's *Bowling Alone*
John Rawls's *Theory of Justice*
Jean-Jacques Rousseau's *The Social Contract*
Theda Skocpol's *States and Social Revolutions*
Adam Smith's *The Wealth of Nations*
Sun Tzu's *The Art of War*
Henry David Thoreau's *Civil Disobedience*
Thucydides's *The History of the Peloponnesian War*
Kenneth Waltz's *Theory of International Politics*
Max Weber's *Politics as a Vocation*
Odd Arne Westad's *The Global Cold War: Third World Interventions And The Making Of Our Times*

POSTCOLONIAL STUDIES

Roland Barthes's *Mythologies*
Frantz Fanon's *Black Skin, White Masks*
Homi K. Bhabha's *The Location of Culture*
Gustavo Gutiérrez's *A Theology of Liberation*
Edward Said's *Orientalism*
Gayatri Chakravorty Spivak's *Can the Subaltern Speak?*

PSYCHOLOGY

Gordon Allport's *The Nature of Prejudice*
Alan Baddeley & Graham Hitch's *Aggression: A Social Learning Analysis*
Albert Bandura's *Aggression: A Social Learning Analysis*
Leon Festinger's *A Theory of Cognitive Dissonance*
Sigmund Freud's *The Interpretation of Dreams*
Betty Friedan's *The Feminine Mystique*
Michael R. Gottfredson & Travis Hirschi's *A General Theory of Crime*
Eric Hoffer's *The True Believer: Thoughts on the Nature of Mass Movements*
William James's *Principles of Psychology*
Elizabeth Loftus's *Eyewitness Testimony*
A. H. Maslow's *A Theory of Human Motivation*
Stanley Milgram's *Obedience to Authority*
Steven Pinker's *The Better Angels of Our Nature*
Oliver Sacks's *The Man Who Mistook His Wife For a Hat*
Richard Thaler & Cass Sunstein's *Nudge: Improving Decisions About Health, Wealth and Happiness*
Amos Tversky's *Judgment under Uncertainty: Heuristics and Biases*
Philip Zimbardo's *The Lucifer Effect*

SCIENCE

Rachel Carson's *Silent Spring*
William Cronon's *Nature's Metropolis: Chicago And The Great West*
Alfred W. Crosby's *The Columbian Exchange*
Charles Darwin's *On the Origin of Species*
Richard Dawkin's *The Selfish Gene*
Thomas Kuhn's *The Structure of Scientific Revolutions*
Geoffrey Parker's *Global Crisis: War, Climate Change and Catastrophe in the Seventeenth Century*
Mathis Wackernagel & William Rees's *Our Ecological Footprint*

SOCIOLOGY

Michelle Alexander's *The New Jim Crow: Mass Incarceration in the Age of Colorblindness*
Gordon Allport's *The Nature of Prejudice*
Albert Bandura's *Aggression: A Social Learning Analysis*
Hanna Batatu's *The Old Social Classes And The Revolutionary Movements Of Iraq*
Ha-Joon Chang's *Kicking Away the Ladder*
W. E. B. Du Bois's *The Souls of Black Folk*
Émile Durkheim's *On Suicide*
Frantz Fanon's *Black Skin, White Masks*
Frantz Fanon's *The Wretched of the Earth*
Eric Foner's *Reconstruction: America's Unfinished Revolution, 1863-1877*
Eugene Genovese's *Roll, Jordan, Roll: The World the Slaves Made*
Jack Goldstone's *Revolution and Rebellion in the Early Modern World*
Antonio Gramsci's *The Prison Notebooks*
Richard Herrnstein & Charles A Murray's *The Bell Curve: Intelligence and Class Structure in American Life*
Eric Hoffer's *The True Believer: Thoughts on the Nature of Mass Movements*
Jane Jacobs's *The Death and Life of Great American Cities*
Robert Lucas's *Why Doesn't Capital Flow from Rich to Poor Countries?*
Jay Macleod's *Ain't No Makin' It: Aspirations and Attainment in a Low Income Neighborhood*
Elaine May's *Homeward Bound: American Families in the Cold War Era*
Douglas McGregor's *The Human Side of Enterprise*
C. Wright Mills's *The Sociological Imagination*

Thomas Piketty's *Capital in the Twenty-First Century*
Robert D. Putman's *Bowling Alone*
David Riesman's *The Lonely Crowd: A Study of the Changing American Character*
Edward Said's *Orientalism*
Joan Wallach Scott's *Gender and the Politics of History*
Theda Skocpol's *States and Social Revolutions*
Max Weber's *The Protestant Ethic and the Spirit of Capitalism*

THEOLOGY

Augustine's *Confessions*
Benedict's *Rule of St Benedict*
Gustavo Gutiérrez's *A Theology of Liberation*
Carole Hillenbrand's *The Crusades: Islamic Perspectives*
David Hume's *Dialogues Concerning Natural Religion*
Immanuel Kant's *Religion within the Boundaries of Mere Reason*
Ernst Kantorowicz's *The King's Two Bodies: A Study in Medieval Political Theology*
Søren Kierkegaard's *The Sickness Unto Death*
C. S. Lewis's *The Abolition of Man*
Saba Mahmood's *The Politics of Piety: The Islamic Revival and the Feminist Subject*
Baruch Spinoza's *Ethics*
Keith Thomas's *Religion and the Decline of Magic*

COMING SOON

Chris Argyris's *The Individual and the Organisation*
Seyla Benhabib's *The Rights of Others*
Walter Benjamin's *The Work Of Art in the Age of Mechanical Reproduction*
John Berger's *Ways of Seeing*
Pierre Bourdieu's *Outline of a Theory of Practice*
Mary Douglas's *Purity and Danger*
Roland Dworkin's *Taking Rights Seriously*
James G. March's *Exploration and Exploitation in Organisational Learning*
Ikujiro Nonaka's *A Dynamic Theory of Organizational Knowledge Creation*
Griselda Pollock's *Vision and Difference*
Amartya Sen's *Inequality Re-Examined*
Susan Sontag's *On Photography*
Yasser Tabbaa's *The Transformation of Islamic Art*
Ludwig von Mises's *Theory of Money and Credit*

Macat Pairs

*Analyse historical and modern issues
from opposite sides of an argument.
Pairs include:*

INTERNATIONAL RELATIONS IN THE 21ST CENTURY

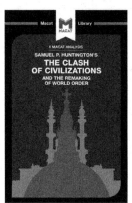

Samuel P. Huntington's
The Clash of Civilisations

In his highly influential 1996 book, Huntington offers a vision of a post-Cold War world in which conflict takes place not between competing ideologies but between cultures. The worst clash, he argues, will be between the Islamic world and the West: the West's arrogance and belief that its culture is a "gift" to the world will come into conflict with Islam's obstinacy and concern that its culture is under attack from a morally decadent "other."

Clash inspired much debate between different political schools of thought. But its greatest impact came in helping define American foreign policy in the wake of the 2001 terrorist attacks in New York and Washington.

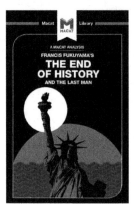

Francis Fukuyama's
The End of History and the Last Man

Published in 1992, *The End of History and the Last Man* argues that capitalist democracy is the final destination for all societies. Fukuyama believed democracy triumphed during the Cold War because it lacks the "fundamental contradictions" inherent in communism and satisfies our yearning for freedom and equality. Democracy therefore marks the endpoint in the evolution of ideology, and so the "end of history." There will still be "events," but no fundamental change in ideology.

Macat analyses are available from all good bookshops and libraries.

Access hundreds of analyses through one, multimedia tool.
Join free for one month **library.macat.com**

Macat Disciplines

Access the greatest ideas and thinkers across entire disciplines, including

MAN AND THE ENVIRONMENT

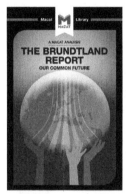
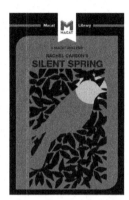
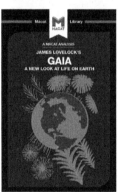
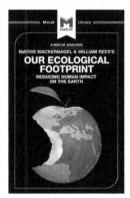

The Brundtland Report's, *Our Common Future*
Rachel Carson's, *Silent Spring*
James Lovelock's, *Gaia: A New Look at Life on Earth*
Mathis Wackernagel & William Rees's, *Our Ecological Footprint*

Macat analyses are available from all good bookshops and libraries.

Access hundreds of analyses through one, multimedia tool.
Join free for one month **library.macat.com**

Printed in the United States
by Baker & Taylor Publisher Services